Emotional, Physical and Sexual Abuse

Giovanni Corona • Emmanuele A. Jannini •
Mario Maggi
Editors

Emotional, Physical and Sexual Abuse

Impact in Children and Social Minorities

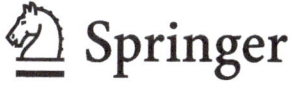

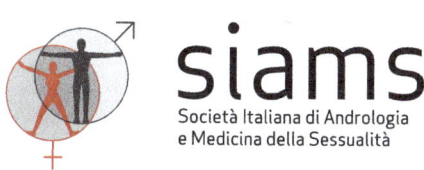

Editors
Giovanni Corona
Endocrinology Unit
Maggiore-Bellaria Hospital
Medical Department
Azienda-Usl Bologna
Bologna, Italy

Emmanuele A. Jannini
Department of System Medicine
University of Rome Tor Vergata
Rome
Italy

Mario Maggi
Sexual Medicine and Andrology Unit
University of Florence
Florence
Italy

ISBN 978-3-319-06786-5   ISBN 978-3-319-06787-2 (eBook)
DOI 10.1007/978-3-319-06787-2
Springer Cham Heidelberg New York Dordrecht London

Library of Congress Control Number: 2014945566

© Springer International Publishing Switzerland 2014
This work is subject to copyright. All rights are reserved by the Publisher, whether the whole or part of the material is concerned, specifically the rights of translation, reprinting, reuse of illustrations, recitation, broadcasting, reproduction on microfilms or in any other physical way, and transmission or information storage and retrieval, electronic adaptation, computer software, or by similar or dissimilar methodology now known or hereafter developed. Exempted from this legal reservation are brief excerpts in connection with reviews or scholarly analysis or material supplied specifically for the purpose of being entered and executed on a computer system, for exclusive use by the purchaser of the work. Duplication of this publication or parts thereof is permitted only under the provisions of the Copyright Law of the Publisher's location, in its current version, and permission for use must always be obtained from Springer. Permissions for use may be obtained through RightsLink at the Copyright Clearance Center. Violations are liable to prosecution under the respective Copyright Law.
The use of general descriptive names, registered names, trademarks, service marks, etc. in this publication does not imply, even in the absence of a specific statement, that such names are exempt from the relevant protective laws and regulations and therefore free for general use.
While the advice and information in this book are believed to be true and accurate at the date of publication, neither the authors nor the editors nor the publisher can accept any legal responsibility for any errors or omissions that may be made. The publisher makes no warranty, express or implied, with respect to the material contained herein.

Printed on acid-free paper

Springer is part of Springer Science+Business Media (www.springer.com)

Preface

Emotional, physical, and sexual abuse may have devastating effects on victims. This is particularly true when victims are socially vulnerable individuals, such as children, disables, or sexual minorities. Emotional and physical abuse has a corrosive impact on mental health and well-being, exacerbating the low self-esteem, poor coping behaviors, and social relationships of individuals. Indeed, sexual abuse when occurring in a crucial period for developing emotion, mature self-representation, personality and social relationship—such as childhood is—may result in severe sexual and mental health disorders.

Prevention of offences towards these vulnerable categories includes social educational plans. However, when offenders suffer from a paraphilic disorder, a comprehensive approach based on psychological and medical treatment (such as hormonal castration) is recommended.

The present book describes the characteristic of maltreatment towards socially frail individuals focusing on both victims and perpetrators aspects. Moreover, it illustrates social and treatment interventions aimed to decrease the recidivism risk of abuse.

Florence, Italy   Alessandra D. Fisher

Contents

1 **Pedophilia** 1
   Abhi Shetty, Ayanangshu Nayak, Ray Travers, Hasit Vaidya,
   and Kevan Wylie

2 **Treatment of Paraphilic Sex Offenders** 17
   Alessandra D. Fisher and Mario Maggi

3 **Negative Attitudes to Lesbians and Gay Men: Persecutors
   and Victims** 33
   Vittorio Lingiardi and Nicola Nardelli

4 **Transphobia** 49
   Elisa Bandini and Mario Maggi

5 **Sexual Abuse and Sexual Function** 61
   Alessandra H. Rellini

6 **Childhood Sexual Abuse and Psychopathology** 71
   Giovanni Castellini, Mario Maggi, and Valdo Ricca

7 **Atypical Sexual Offenders** 93
   Daniele Mollaioli, Erika Limoncin, Giacomo Ciocca,
   and Emmanuele A. Jannini

Index 111

Pedophilia

Abhi Shetty, Ayanangshu Nayak, Ray Travers, Hasit Vaidya, and Kevan Wylie

1.1 Introduction

Very few topics of public debate evoke as many feelings of revulsion and moral disgust as pedophilia. Practising clinicians are not immune from such reactions. Public perception is influenced by media stories of pedophile rings, extreme abuse, maltreatment and significant harm including murder of children by adults who also had sexual contact with them. It is hence important to distinguish pedophilia from pedophilic disorder as defined by the Diagnostic and Statistical Manual of Mental Disorders Fifth Edition (DSM-5) [1] and differentiate this from child sexual abuse which is focused on harm caused to the child [2].

Pedophilia and pedophilic disorder are psychiatric diagnoses according to the International Statistical Classification of Diseases and Related Health Problems 10th Revision (ICD-10) and DSM-5, respectively. It is categorised as a "disorder of adult personality and behaviour" in the ICD-10 under the subcategory of "disorder of sexual preference" [3]. ICD-10 defines it as a sexual preference for children, boys or girls or both, usually of prepubertal or early pubertal age [3]. DSM-5 classifies this as a paraphilic disorder (i.e. sexual preference disorder) and confines the sexual preference in pedophilia to prepubertal children only and defines this as children generally aged 13 years or younger [1].

This chapter aims to describe various characteristics of this paraphilic disorder including its definition, subtypes, current diagnostic criteria, gender bias, onset and course, epidemiology, aetiology and its assessment. As pedophilia is closely associated with crimes against children as well as significant public stigma especially in recent times this aspect will also be briefly explored. Fictionalised case vignettes will be presented to illustrate the problem further. Therapeutic concerns will be addressed in the next chapter. The consequences of child sexual abuse are addressed in subsequent chapters.

Much of what we know about pedophilia is through studies of clinical populations particularly of child sexual offenders in prison or forensic settings. Most of these studies involve men only and have relatively small sample sizes. As noted by Quinsey (1986), identified pedophile offenders are almost always male. Almost nothing is written about women who commit incestuous and non-incestuous sex crimes [4]. There are some population-based surveys based on anonymous responses from predominantly male college students but some have female respondents as well. Hence any scientific discourse on pedophilia is essentially limited by its lack of generalisability. It also suffers from minimisation and concealment bias due to potential stigma and fear of self-incrimination among study respondents.

1.2 Definition, Subtypes and Diagnostic Criteria

Krafft-Ebing's *Psychopathia Sexualis* in 1886 was one of the early publications where pedophilia as a diagnostic terminology was mentioned (*pedophilia erotica*) [5]. He had classified pedophilia as a "sexual perversion" based on non-procreational nature of the sexual contact [5]. This Victorian medical psychopathology constructed a male figure driven by forces beyond his control. It did not place a female voice in the narrative [6]. One part of his case definition, however, survives to this day as a central feature of this condition, namely, that it is a sexual preference disorder. DSM-5 reminds the reader that Paraphilic Disorders occur almost exclusively in men [1]. DSM-5 retains the diagnostic criteria of DSM-IV-TR [7] but makes the important distinction between pedophilic disorder from pedophilic sexual interest only (satisfying Criterion A only in Table 1.1) [1]. Currently, all three parameters (Criteria A, B and C in Table 1.1) have to be fulfilled for the diagnosis of a pedophilic disorder. Individuals who have predominant or marked sexual interest in children but do not show any subjective or objective evidence of personal distress, of functional limitation or of having acted on their interests are now not considered to be mentally ill but to have a pedophilic sexual orientation [1].

Both ICD-10 and DSM-5 criteria for this condition are not without controversies. Much of the debate has focused on distinguishing mental disorder from illegal or immoral behaviour [8]. Most individuals with pedophilia do not voluntarily seek

Table 1.1 Diagnostic criteria for pedophilic disorder in DSM-5 (302.2) [1, pp. 697–698] (reproduced with permission)

(A) Over a period of at least 6 months, recurrent, intense sexually arousing fantasies, sexual urges, or behaviours involving sexual activity with a prepubescent child or children (generally age 13 years or younger)

(B) The individual has acted on these sexual urges, or the sexual urges or fantasies cause marked distress or interpersonal difficulty

(C) The individual is at least age 16 years and at least 5 years older than the child or children in Criterion A.

Note: Do not include an individual in late adolescence involved in an ongoing sexual relationship with a 12- or 13-year-old

Specify whether:
   Exclusive type (attracted only to children)
   Nonexclusive type

Specify if:
   Sexually attracted to males
   Sexually attracted to females
   Sexually attracted to both

Specify if:
   Limited to incest

treatment due to distress or functional impairment. They often come in contact with mental health services following referral from the criminal justice system due to sexual offences against children. Courts deal with women differently. They are rarely charged with sex offences other than prostitution and sexual abuse by women appears to be a vastly underreported crime [9]. Pathologising criminal behaviour risks psychiatry being seen as society's moral police.

There is a further criticism about the age of children associated with pedophilic urges, fantasies or acts. ICD-10 criteria includes "a sexual preference for children, usually of prepubertal or early pubertal age" [3, p. 171], whereas DSM 5 classifies children aged 13 or under as prepubescent children and limits its definition to include such children only [1]. There is considerable evidence that the age of puberty has steadily fallen in many societies or countries over the last 150 years. [10]. As a result, prepubescent would exclude a large number of children in contemporary society. There is evidence to suggest that some men are exclusively or preferentially sexually attracted to pubescent children corresponding to Tanner stages 2 and 3 [11]. This is not known to be the case for some women. Hebephilia is a term coined by Gluek in 1955 to define such individuals' sexual preference [11]. The Paraphilias Subworkgroup for DSM-5 therefore proposed replacing pedophilic disorder with *pedohebephilic disorder*, either *pedophilic*, *hebephilic* or *pedohebephilic* subtype; however, this was not considered in the final publication of DSM-5 [11]. The term infantophilia has been used to identify individuals who are preferentially sexually attracted to children younger than 5 years of age; however, this is not recognised in the major classificatory systems [12].

DSM criteria for pedophilia have not been adequately field tested and many clinicians outside of the USA rarely use these criteria in their practice which brings into question the usefulness of the current diagnostic criteria [13].

1.3 Onset and Course

A significant number of child sex offenders report an early onset of sexual fantasies, sexual interest and sexual curiosity involving children. Freund and Kuban (1993) compared 76 child sex offenders with 78 male college students and found that a higher proportion of men with pedophilia reported curiosity about seeing children in the nude as young adolescents whilst the healthy controls lost this curiosity by puberty [14]. Among a sample of 129 child sex offenders Marshal et al. (1991) reported an onset of pedophilic fantasies prior to the age of 20 in 41 % of non-incest offenders who molested boys; overall 29 % self-reported an early onset of pedophilic fantasies [15]. In the USA the National Incident-Based Reporting System (NIBRS) reported a 40 % sexual assault rate against children younger than 12 years by juveniles who were most frequently 14 years old [16]. In a large population-based study of 16,109 adults who were sexual offenders Abel and Harlow (2001) identified 4,007 child molesters and found that 40 % of pedophilic child molesters had acted on their fantasies before the age of 15 and the majority by the age of 20 [17]. Studies of this kind are not available for female sexual offenders. Women are under-represented and under-reported for a variety of reasons [18].

In a study of 168 sex offenders Dickey et al. (2002) found that pedophilic offenders were more likely to re-offend even after the age of 40 compared to rape and sexual sadism offenders; men with pedophilia comprised 60 % of all older offenders [19]. Other studies have found long-term sexual recidivism among child offenders although it is unclear how many of these were diagnosed with pedophilia [20, 21]. There are no empirical studies which have looked at the long-term course of pedophilia. However systematic reviews of various psychological, social and pharmacological treatment interventions for pedophilic child offenders indicate poor evidence of efficacy [22, 23]. Most researchers agree that while the behavioural manifestations can be modified to a certain extent the underlying sexual preference remains stable long term [12, 24].

DSM-5 acknowledges the development of pedophilic sexual attraction around the onset of puberty, a lifelong course and the age-related reduction in the frequency of sexual behaviour directed towards children and compares this with normal sexual development and behaviour [1]. Seto (2012) argues whether pedophilia can be considered a variant of sexual orientation based on age similar to heterosexuality and homosexuality which are based on gender [25]. Other commentators have supported this theory [12]. Whilst highlighting the extreme asymmetry of any sexual interaction between an adult and a child which is appropriately criminalised, Seto (2012) also advocates for reducing stigma to enable help seeking behaviour by people with pedophilia [25].

1.4 Epidemiology

True population prevalence of pedophilia is unknown as such studies have not been conducted. In a male undergraduate sample of 193, Briere and Runtz (1989) found that 21 % had reported sexual attraction to small children (age and gender unspecified) [26]. In the same study 9 % admitted to having child-focused sexual fantasies and 5 % masturbating to such fantasies. 7 % actually reported an inclination to having sex with a child provided they are not detected and punished [26]. In a much larger survey of 582 male college students 3 % admitted to having any sexual experience with a child [27]. Rates of 3–5 % have also been reported in similar smaller surveys [28] and DSM-5 uses these rates as an estimate of the higher end of population prevalence [1].

Men account for the majority of the identified people with pedophilia. Estimates vary from 90 % to 99 % [12, 17]. In The Abel and Harlow Child Molestation Prevention Study (2001) 65 % of the 4,007 child molesters fit the diagnostic criteria for pedophilia, but they estimate that a higher proportion could be missed due to under or inconsistent reporting [17]. They found that offenders with pedophilia on average molest four times the number of children and commit 10 times more sexual acts against children than non-pedophilic child offenders [17]. There are significant variations in the reported demographic characteristics of pedophiles compared to the general population [24]; however, Abel and Harlow (2001) in their large study of child molesters found that their sample matched the general US population in terms of ethnicity, socio-economic status, education, marital status and religiosity [17].

Many studies report a higher prevalence of homosexuality and bisexuality among men with pedophilia [12]. There are some significant differences reported in the literature between men who sexually offend against boys compared to girls which are highlighted in Table 1.2 [29].

People with pedophilia might be attracted exclusively to children or to adults as well. Abel and Harlow (2001) reported only 7 % exclusive pedophilia sufferers in their study [17]. The manifestation of pedophilia can be confined to sexual urges and fantasies to non-contact acts and sexual touching. Vaginal, anal or oral penetration and the use of force are rare [12, 24]. Non-contact sexual behaviour can involve peeping at nude or semi-nude children and exposing themselves or masturbating in the presence of children. All of the above can move on to much more intrusive physical contact including unsolicited genital rubbing against a child, sexualised touching through the clothes as well as in the nude and occasionally engaging in oral sex or anal and vaginal penetration [12, 24]. Extreme violence and sexual brutality which often get publicised in the media are fortunately extremely rare [24]. However co-morbidity with other paraphilias is in fact quite common unlike previously thought with an estimated 50–70 % of pedophiles also fulfilling the diagnostic criteria for voyeurism, exhibitionism, frotteurism or sadism [12, 30].

Pedophilic incest offenders are most likely to use physical force and subject children to penetrative intercourse [31]. Prevalence rates of incest and intrafamilial

Table 1.2 Comparison of heterosexual and homosexual men with pedophilia [29, p. 311]. Reproduced with permission

Heterosexual men with pedophilia	Homosexual men with pedophilia
Few victims	Many victims (up to hundreds)
Offences repeated with same victim for months/years	Offences commonly occur only once with same victim
Offences occur in victim's home	Offences occur away from victim's home
Mean age of victim is 8 years	Mean age of victim is 10 years
Offender attracted to adult women	Offender not sexually attracted to adults of either sex
Offender commonly married	Offender single
Behaviour commenced in adulthood	Behaviour commenced in adolescence
Often low socio-economic class, unemployed, alcoholic, lower IQ, psychopathic	Stable/employed, average IQ but "immature": prefers company of children, not interested in friendships with adults

offenders range from 27 % to 68 % [16, 17] and one study reported a significant overlap between intrafamilial and extrafamilial child offenders [32]. Girls are twice as likely as boys to have been victims of unwanted sexual contact in childhood as recalled by adult respondents [24]. Able and Harlow (2001) assert that pedophilia is the single most common cause of child sexual abuse; people with pedophilia are responsible for 88 % of child molestations in the USA and 95 % of sexual acts against children [17].

Use of child pornography both online and offline including images, videos, chat rooms and sexual grooming are significant recent concerns which have received attention [33, 34]. Amongst child sexual offenders, those who use child pornography are more likely to have pedophilia [34]. In fact, extensive use of child pornography has been specifically acknowledged in the DSM-5 as a helpful diagnostic indicator of pedophilic disorder [1]. While some studies have reported a high rate of contact sexual offence against children amongst child pornography users, Eke et al. (2011) found only 4 % of the 541 men registered for child pornography offences went on to commit a new contact child sex offence, 2 % were later identified to have committed historical contact sex offences and 7 % were charged for new child pornography offences [33].

1.5 Female Pedophilia

As has been described earlier available research on female pedophilia is limited. Crassiati (1998) has highlighted how ambiguities in conceptualising sexual abuse by women, other than in relatively clear-cut cases of indecent assault and incest, seem to contribute to difficulties in thinking about, identifying and investigating female pedophilia [35]. A recent study that attempted to classify female pedophilic inclinations noted three groups: those women who targeted young children or adolescent children or those coerced into sexual abuse by men [36].

Meyer (1992) notes that there are similarities and differences between female and male perpetrators (i.e. defences used, power dynamics, objectification of victims, histories involving sexual victimisation in childhood, etc.) [18]. Women can carry out all forms of sexual abuse of children. 29 of the 52 women involved in Saradjian's study (1996) admitted becoming sexually aroused to thoughts of sexual acts which cause physical pain to children [36].

1.6 Aetiology

The cause of pedophilia is unknown. A number of theories have been put forward to explain its prevalence. Psychoanalytic thinking was very influential in the early part of the twentieth century; however, this was gradually replaced by cognitive and behavioural approaches. In recent times a number of neuropsychiatric studies have been carried out indicating differences between pedophilic and non-pedophilic men. To the authors' knowledge to date no such work has been completed on women.

1.6.1 Neuropsychiatric Differences

Kraft-Ebbing conceptualised pedophilia as a disease of the brain [4].The frontal lobe is involved in reflecting, planning and conscious inhibition of sexual desire and behaviour whilst sexual arousal to various stimuli is primarily mediated in the temporal cortex [37]. The cerebellum also has an important role to play in learning and modulating behaviour [38]. In a sample of 18 men with pedophilia from a high security prison Schiffer et al. (2007) found decreased grey matter volume in the ventral striatum, orbitofrontal cortex and the cerebellum compared to healthy matched controls using structural magnetic resonance imaging (MRI) [39]. Using functional imaging techniques Cohen et al. (2002) reported reduced glucose metabolism in the right inferior temporal cortex and the superior ventral frontal gyrus in a small sample of seven men with pedophilia compared to the control sample [37]. These findings can be compared with the neuropathological findings in other impulse control disorders like obsessive–compulsive disorder (OCD), antisocial personality and addictions [39]. Cohen et al. (2002) link high incidence of childhood sexual abuse in their study sample as a causative factor in neurodevelopmental abnormalities; however, the direction of causality as well as other confounding factors are not clear [37]. These results though have not been replicated in other studies [24]. For example, Cantor et al. (2008) compared structural MRI findings between 65 pedophilic men with 63 controls and reported a lack of difference in grey matter volumes in the frontal and temporal regions but significant differences in the white matter volume in the superior orbito-frontal and right arcuate fasciculi [40]. Dysregulation in the brain monoamine system (serotonin, dopamine and norepinephrine) has also been proposed as a candidate theory for pedophilia [12, 22].

Acquired brain lesions have been implicated in the onset of pedophilia later in life [24]. There is a higher incidence of head injury associated with unconsciousness before the age of 13 among pedophilic sex offenders [41]. Other neuropsychological and physical differences have also been reported among pedophilic sex offenders including lower intelligence quotient (IQ) scores, impairment in memory tests, poor educational attainment, short stature and left handedness [42, 43]. Lower intelligence was positively correlated with lower age of child victims [43].

1.6.2 Psychosocial Differences

Pedophilic sexual offenders are more likely to be victims of sexual abuse in childhood themselves than non-pedophilic sexual offenders [12, 24, 32]. Jesperson et al. (2009) conducted a meta-analysis of 17 studies comparing rates of various types of abuse history among 1,037 sex offenders with 1,762 non-sex offenders and found a higher prevalence of sexual abuse history among sex offenders and significantly higher prevalence in pedophilic sex offenders [44]. The victim age preference of pedophilic offenders was similar to the age when they were abused in childhood [45]. Psychoanalysts have used these findings to theorise that individuals with pedophila are "stuck" in an earlier stage of psychosexual development due to childhood trauma and start identifying with the aggressor and hence perpetuate the cycle of abuse [12, 24, 32]. Behavioural theorists postulate that individuals with pedophilia are conditioned by early childhood sexual experiences including of early abuse to develop paraphilic sexual arousal patterns [12, 24].

Motz (2008) theorised that women who sexually abuse their children treat them as narcissistic extensions of themselves and inflict violence on them in a perverse attempt to rid themselves of underlying feelings of inadequacy, guilt and depression [46]. The sexual interaction, whilst often misunderstood by clinicians, provides a temporary release from these feelings, an escape from their self-loathing and unhappiness, but after an initial euphoria the depression and guilt return and a vicious cycle is established [46].

These results should be interpreted cautiously as most victims of childhood sexual abuse do not go on to abuse children in adulthood [24] and non-clinical samples have not shown differences in sexual abuse history between individuals who have had sexual contact with children compared to those who deny such contact [27].

Parental neglect, attachment difficulties, maternal mental illness, hyper sexuality, deficits in empathy, poor social skills, emotional dysregulation, impulsivity and predilection to aggressive behaviour are more likely to be associated with individuals with pedophilia who tend to act out their pedophilic fantasies [47]. Stress, drug and alcohol intoxication are contextual factors which are more likely to increase the risk of sexual offending against children [47]. See Ward and beech (2006) for a review of the various etiological factors associated with pedophilia and an integrated approach to understanding sexual offending against children [47].

1.7 Social and Legal Perspectives

Pedophilia has generated an increased level of controversy in recent years. With the advent of the Internet and increased connectedness, media stories of national or international police operations targeting pedophile rings have not been uncommon in the last 25 years [48].

In many cases these high-profile law enforcement operations have been against well-organised network of people engaged in direct sexual contact with children or adolescents. In other cases the targeted people have traded in pornographic images of children. Recently, many media celebrities in the UK have faced allegations of child sexual abuse [49].

Invariably, these cases have generated widespread public anxiety even though there are examples of balanced reporting [50]. The media have played an active role in shaping public opinion. Megan's Law in the USA and Sarah's Law in the UK are well-known examples of this trend [51].

In response to widespread concerns many countries have chosen to tighten laws against child sexual abuse. Very few systematic studies have investigated this trend across national boundaries. Sociologists Frank et al. (2010) report a general tightening of laws in this area in majority of countries from 1945 to 2005, most of these in the second half of this period studied [52]. They postulate that the trend is part of a wider social phenomenon whereby individual freedom is highly valued and hence consent issues have become paramount in sexual relationships [52]. In most countries age of consent for sexual intercourse is between the ages of 14 and 18.

Historian Fass (2003) hypothesises that as the pace of change in almost every society has increased due to globalisation, general anxiety about such changes is displaced to the symbolically sensitive area about our concern for protection of children [53]. Law enforcement agencies have responded to such changes in the social outlook by tightening not just the laws but also procedures in dealing with these cases. For instance, in the UK, the Crown Prosecution Service recently updated their guidelines to individual police forces in the country dealing with allegations of child sexual abuse [54].

1.8 Assessment

A thorough psychiatric history should be obtained for any patient presenting with suspected pedophilia. Table 1.3 lists psychological co-morbid conditions which are associated with pedophilia [30, 55–57]. Some of these conditions could be psychological consequences of the pedophilic orientation and its associated psychosocial or legal difficulties.

Wherever co-morbid psychiatric conditions are present their relationship to pedophilia or pedophilic behaviour should be clarified. For example, it is possible to envisage that for some individuals acting out pedophilic thoughts or fantasies could only happen during hypomanic or inebriated periods. Similarly, onset of these conditions could also shed light on the possible interrelationships of these

Table 1.3 Psychological co-morbidity associated with pedophilia [30, 55–57]

OCD
Anxiety disorders
Dysthymia and depressive disorders
Manic or hypomanic episode
Conduct disorder
Antisocial personality disorder
Borderline personality disorder and other impulse control disorders
Narcissistic personality disorder
Mental retardation
Alcohol or other psychoactive substance abuse
Adjustment disorders
Other paraphilias

conditions [58]. The psychiatric history should also include detailed personal history. This should incorporate any developmental adversity such as head injury, delayed milestones, history of any form of abuse or evidence of insecure attachment.

Detailed psychosexual history is another essential element in the assessment of suspected individuals with pedophilia. Any indicator of hypersexuality should be noted. Both sexual thoughts and behaviours should be evaluated. In the presence of any paraphilias, any fantasy should be carefully evaluated noting circumstances where acting out becomes more likely. Assessments of mental illness, psychological health and psychosexual functioning should incorporate information available from other sources besides self-reports. Other types of paraphilias such as sadomasochistic fantasies or behaviours should be given special emphasis due to risk implications [24].

A physical examination and blood investigations including endocrine investigations should form part of a standard medical assessment of the patient presenting with suspected pedophilia. There is very little practical use of endocrine measures in the diagnosis of pedophilia, but baseline hormone levels should still be carried out for comparison in case chemical castration as a treatment for child sex offenders is planned.

1.9 Psychophysiological Assessments

In addition to clinical and psychological assessments psychophysiological assessment tools such as Penile Plethysmography (PPG) or Viewing Time (VT) complement clinical assessment in the diagnosis of pedophilia as self-reported denial is very high amongst patients presenting with child sex abuse. Of these PPG is the best validated tool.

1.9.1 PPG

It is assumed that in men sexual arousal is accompanied by an increase of penile circumference or volume. Harris et al. (1996) reported a relationship between self-reported sexual arousal in non-offending men exposed to sexually stimulating visual or auditory cues and their penile circumference or volume [59]. Furthermore, they reported even more discriminating difference between pedophilic offenders and non-offenders when the stimuli used are auditory or visual cues using children [59]. PPG can be used in adolescent offender population as well [60]. PPG sensitivity is variable depending on the centre as well as the group targeted but usually varies between 60 and 86 % [57]. The specificity similarly varies between 80 % and over 90 % except in adolescents where sensitivity reported is as low as 40 % [57]. PPG can not only help in identifying sexual preference towards children but also other paraphilias including motivation towards coercion and violence [57]. Lalumiere et al. (2003) reviewed effectiveness of PPG in different areas and found that its accuracy can be increased by adding a semantic task to make sure that the participant engages with the cues [61]. PPG is controversial as child pornographic images may be illegal to store in some jurisdiction apart from obvious ethical issues about its use in subjects accused of sexual offences; it is not useful in females; its effectiveness is dependent on the absence of erectile dysfunction; it is also an invasive and expensive procedure [12].

1.9.2 VT

This test depends on the preference patterns of different groups of child molesters viewing various images, and a recent study by Leuterneu (2002) has highlighted its merits and demerits in relation to PPG and reported that VT was better able to identify child sex offenders attracted to girls and equally effective in identifying offenders attracted to boys [62]. Abel Assessment for Sexual Interest (AASI) is a self-report questionnaire and also assesses viewing times to computer-based images [63].

Other physiological or psychological measures such as penile temperature, blood pressure, scales and card sorts, Implicit Association Test as well as Screening Scale for Pedophilic Interest (SSPI) have been used for diagnostic purposes [57].

1.9.3 Risk Assessment

Detailed risk assessment of child sexual offence is beyond the scope of this chapter. However, clinical and psychophysiological assessments contribute greatly towards risk assessment as pedophilia is a strong risk factor towards child sexual offences. They are important discriminators in terms of dynamic risk factors. Various standard risk instruments such as STATIC-99 or SORAG can be used for measuring static risk factors [24].

1.10 Fictionalised Case Vignettes

1.10.1 Vignette 1

Mr X is a 62-year-old man with mild learning disability and antisocial personality traits. When 23 he was arrested and subsequently sent to a low secure hospital detained under the Mental Health Act. Prior to his arrest he was living with his wife of 2 years and her three young children—two boys aged 7 and 12 and a girl aged 15. He was unemployed and had an alcohol problem.

The index offence related to penetrative anal intercourse that he subjected his 7-year-old stepson to when intoxicated with alcohol. He was caught during the act and reported to the police by his wife. He had also threatened her and the distressed boy with a knife when she tried to intervene. During his trial two previous convictions for indecent exposure to school children came to light when he was in his late teens. He also revealed that he was sexually abused by his maternal uncle between the ages of 7 and 13. All three stepchildren testified to unwanted sexual touching and gazing by Mr X in the previous 2 years.

The AASI test revealed his viewing time was highest for both pubescent and prepubescent children of both sexes. He has been observed flicking through children's section of shopping catalogues and trying to secrete pictures by staff during day leave. He has also been noted to track children in public toilets. However, he has consistently denied sexual interest in children. He has shown deficits in empathy, remorse and emotional expression and his engagement with staff has been very superficial. He has spent the last 39 years incarcerated in the secure hospital as he is still deemed to be a risk to children's safety.

1.10.2 Vignette 2

Mr Y is a 21-year-old university student studying computer science. He is single and has come back to live with his parents after an episode of severe depression when he had to take time off his course. Over the past year he has increasingly isolated himself from his peers, found it difficult to concentrate on his studies and took to excessive cannabis use.

Both his parents are high achievers in the academic world. He is the only child. Although academically bright he has always felt short of meeting his parent's expectations. When he was 12 he was sexually assaulted by an unknown man in the school library. He never reported this crime but has carried feelings of guilt ever since. He also developed symptoms suggestive of post-traumatic stress disorder and refused to go to school. He was home schooled for the next 2 years by his mother following which he was able to reintegrate into mainstream schooling.

However, soon after returning home he made a significant suicide attempt by taking an overdose of his antidepressants. He was admitted to a psychiatric ward and over the next 2 months gradually started revealing to his therapist that he was sexually attracted to adolescent girls and had for the first time accessed indecent images of young girls online just prior to the suicide attempt. He had become convinced that he had been found out by the police and hence had tried to kill himself.

Conclusion

Pedophilia is a complex condition of unknown aetiology. It seems to affect a small proportion of the population who are predominantly men with heterogeneous socio-demographic profile. However, pedophilia can have profound negative impact on the sufferer, the children they come into contact with and society in general. Good quality research in this area is limited and hence needs to be pursued to improve our understanding further.

References

1. American Psychiatric Association (2013) Diagnostic and statistical manual of mental disorders DSM-5. American Psychiatric Press, Washington, DC
2. Hillberg T, Hamilton-Giachritsis C, Dixon L (2011) Review of meta-analyses on the association between child sexual abuse and adult mental health difficulties: a systematic approach. Trauma Violence Abuse 12(1):38–49
3. World Health Organization (2010) International statistical classification of diseases and related health problems, 10th revision. http://apps.who.int/classifications/icd10/browse/2010/en. Accessed 29 Jan 2014
4. Quinsey VL (1986) Men who have sex with children. In: Weisstub D (ed) Law and mental health, vol 2. Pergamon, Oxford, pp 532–534
5. Krafft-Ebing R (1965) Psychopathia sexualis with special reference to the antipathic sexual instinct: a medico-forensic study. Paperback Library, New York, NY (Original work published 1886)
6. Walkowitz J (1994) City of dreadful delight. Virago, London
7. American Psychiatric Association (2000) Diagnostic and statistical manual of mental disorders, 4th edn, text rev. American Psychiatric Press, Washington, DC
8. De Block A, Adriaens PR (2013) Pathologizing sexual deviance: a history. J Sex Res 50(3–4):276–298
9. Ford H (2006) Women who sexually abuse children. Wiley, Chichester
10. Bellis MA, Downing J, Ashton JA (2006) Adults at 12? Trends in puberty and their public health consequences. J Epidemiol Community Health 60:910–911
11. Blanchard R (2013) A dissenting opinion on DSM-5 pedophilic disorder. Arch Sex Behav 42:675–678
12. Hall RCW, Hall RCW (2007) A profile of pedophilia: definition, characteristics of offenders, recidivism, treatment outcomes, and forensic issues. Mayo Clin Proc 82(4):457–471
13. Feelgood S, Hoyer J (2008) Child molester or paedophile? Sociolegal versus psychopathological classification of sexual offenders against children. Journal of Sexual Aggression 14(1):33–43
14. Freund K, Kuban M (1993) Toward a testable developmental model of pedophilia: the development of erotic age preference. Child Abuse Negl 17:315–324
15. Marshall WL, Barbaree HE, Eccles A (1991) Early onset and deviant sexuality in child molesters. J Interpers Violence 6:323–336
16. Snyder HN (2000) Sexual assault of young children as reported to law enforcement: victim, incident, and offender characteristics. US Department of Justice, Bureau of Justice Statistics, Washington, DC

17. Abel GG, Harlow N (2001) The Abel and Harlow child molestation prevention study. Excerpted from The Stop Child Molestation Book. Xlibris, Philadelphia, PA. http://www.childmolestationprevention.org/pdfs/study.pdf. Accessed 29 Jan 2014
18. Mayer A (1992) Women sex offenders: treatment and dynamics. Learning Publications, Holmes Beach
19. Dickey R, Nussbaum D, Chevolleau K et al (2002) Age as a differential characteristic of rapists, pedophiles, and sexual sadists. J Sex Marital Ther 28:211–218
20. Hanson RK, Steffy RA, Gauthier R (1993) Long-term recidivism of child molesters. J Consult Clin Psychol 61:646–652
21. Greenberg DM (1998) Sexual recidivism in sex offenders. Can J Psychiatry 43(5):459–465
22. Thibaut F, La Barra F, Gordon H et al (2010) The World Federation of Societies of Biological Psychiatry (WFSBP) guidelines for the biological treatment of paraphilias. World J Biol Psychiatry 11:604–655
23. Långström N, Enebrink P, Laurén EM et al (2013) Preventing sexual abusers of children from reoffending: systematic review of medical and psychological interventions. BMJ. doi:10.1136/bmj.f4630
24. Seto MC (2008) Pedophilia and sexual offending against children: theory, assessment and intervention. American Psychological Association, Washington, DC
25. Seto MC (2012) Is pedophilia a sexual orientation? Arch Sex Behav 41:231–236
26. Briere J, Runtz M (1989) University males' sexual interest in children: predicting potential indices of "pedophilia" in a nonforensic sample. Child Abuse Negl 13(1):65–75
27. Fromuth ME, Burkhart BR, Jones CW (1991) Hidden child molestation: an investigation of adolescent perpetrators in a nonclinical sample. J Interpers Violence 6:376–384
28. McConaghy N (1998) Paedophilia: a review of the evidence. Aust N Z J Psychiatry 32(2):252–265
29. McConaghy N (1993) Sexual behavior: problems and management. Plenum, New York, NY
30. Abel GG, Becker JV, Cunningham-Rathner J et al (1988) Multiple paraphilic diagnoses among sex offenders. Bull Am Acad Psychiatry Law 16:153–168
31. Cohen LJ, Galynker II (2002) Clinical features of pedophilia and implications for treatment. J Psychiatr Pract 8(5):276–289
32. Glasser M, Kolvin I, Campbell D et al (2001) Cycle of child sexual abuse: links between being a victim and becoming a perpetrator. Br J Psychiatry 179:482–494
33. Eke AW, Seto MC, Williams J (2011) Examining the criminal history and future offending of child pornography offenders: an extended prospective follow-up study. Law Hum Behav 35(6):466–478
34. Seto MC, Cantor JM, Blanchard R (2006) Child pornography offenses are a valid diagnostic indicator of pedophilia. J Abnorm Psychol 115:610–615
35. Craissati J (1998) Child sexual abusers: a community treatment approach. Psychology Press, Hove
36. Saradjian J (1996) Women who sexually abuse children. Wiley, Chichester
37. Cohen LJ, Nikiforov K, Gans S et al (2002) Heterosexual male perpetrators of childhood sexual abuse: a preliminary neuropsychiatric model. Psychiatr Q 73:313–336
38. Doya K (2000) Complementary roles of basal ganglia and cerebellum in learning and motor control. Curr Opin Neurobiol 10(6):732–739
39. Schiffer B, Peschel T, Paul T et al (2007) Structural brain abnormalities in the frontostriatal system and cerebellum in pedophilia. J Psychiatr Res 41(9):753–762
40. Cantor JM, Kabani N, Christensen BK et al (2008) Cerebral white matter deficiencies in pedophilic men. J Psychiatr Res 42:167–183
41. Blanchard R, Christensen BK, Strong SM et al (2002) Retrospective self-reports of childhood accidents causing unconsciousness in phallometrically diagnosed pedophiles. Arch Sex Behav 31:511–526
42. Cantor JM, Blanchard R, Robichaud LK et al (2005) Quantitative reanalysis of aggregate data on IQ in sexual offenders. Psychol Bull 131:555–568

43. Cantor JM, Blanchard R, Christensen BK et al (2004) Intelligence, memory, and handedness in pedophilia. Neuropsychology 18(1):3–14
44. Jespersen AF, Lalumiere ML, Seto MC (2009) Sexual abuse history among adult sex offenders and non-sex offenders: a meta-analysis. Child Abuse Negl 33(3):179–192
45. Greenberg DM, Bradford JM, Curry S (1993) A comparison of sexual victimization in the childhoods of pedophiles and hebephiles. J Forensic Sci 38:432–436
46. Motz A (2008) The psychology of female violence: crimes against the body. Routledge, East Sussex
47. Ward T, Beech T (2006) An integrated theory of sexual offending. Aggress Violent Behav 11: 44–63
48. Casciani D (2011) 'World's largest paedophile ring' uncovered. BBC. http://www.bbc.co.uk/news/uk-12762333. Accessed 31 Jan 2014
49. Boffey D (2014) Revealed: how Jimmy Savile abused up to 1,000 victims on BBC premises. The Observer. http://www.theguardian.com/media/2014/jan/18/jimmy-savile-abused-1000-victims-bbc. Accessed 31 Jan 2014
50. Henley J (2013) Paedophilia: bringing dark desires to light. The Guardian. http://www.theguardian.com/society/2013/jan/03/paedophilia-bringing-dark-desires-light. Accessed 31 Jan 2014
51. BBC (2000) To name and shame. BBC. http://news.bbc.co.uk/1/hi/uk/848759.stm. Accessed 31 Jan 2014
52. Frank DJ, Camp BJ, Boutcher SA (2010) Worldwide trend in criminal regulation of sex, 1945–2005. Am Sociol Rev 75(6):867–893
53. Fass PS (2003) Children and globalization. J Soc Hist 36(4):963–977
54. Crown Prosecution Service (2013) Guidelines on prosecuting cases of child sexual abuse. CPS. http://www.cps.gov.uk/legal/a_to_c/child_sexual_abuse/. Accessed 31 Jan 2014
55. Raymond NC, Coleman E, Ohlerking F et al (1999) Psychiatric comorbidity in pedophilic sex offenders. Am J Psychiatry 156:786–788
56. Galli V, McElroy SL, Soutullo CA et al (1999) The psychiatric diagnoses of twenty-two adolescents who have sexually molested other children. Compr Psychiatry 40:85–88
57. Camilleri JA, Quincey VL (2008) Pedophilia assessment and treatment. In: Laws DR, O'Donohue WT (eds) Sexual deviance: theory, assessment, and treatment. The Guildford, New York, NY, pp 183–212
58. Baker M, White T (2002) Sex offenders in high security care in Scotland. J Forensic Psychiatr 13:285–297
59. Harris GT, Rice ME, Quinsey VL et al (1996) Viewing time as a measure of sexual interest among child molesters and normal heterosexual men. Behav Res Ther 34:389–394
60. Seto MC, Lalumière ML, Blanchard R (2000) The discriminative validity of a phallometric test for pedophilic interests among adolescent sex offenders against children. Psychol Assess 12(3):319–327
61. Lalumière ML, Quinsey VL, Harris GT et al (2003) Are rapists differentially aroused by coercive sex in phallometric assessments? Ann NY Acad Sci 989:211–224
62. Letourneau EJ (2002) A comparison of objective measures of sexual arousal and interest: visual reaction time and penile plethysmography. Sex Abuse 14:207–223
63. Abel GG, Jordan A, Hand CG et al (2001) Classification models of child molesters utilizing the Abel Assessment for sexual interest. Child Abuse Negl 25:703–718

Treatment of Paraphilic Sex Offenders

2

Alessandra D. Fisher and Mario Maggi

2.1 Background

2.1.1 Paraphilic Disorder

According to the Diagnostic and Statistical Manual of Mental Disorders (DSM 5) [1] paraphilia is described as any intense and persistent sexual interest other than sexual interest in genital stimulation or preparatory fondling with phenotypically normal, physically mature, consenting human partners. On the other hand, a paraphilic disorder is a paraphilia that is currently causing distress or impairment to the individual or a paraphilia when satisfaction of which entails personal harm or risk of harm to others. In fact, to further define the line between an atypical sexual interest and disorder, the DSM 5 Work Group differentiated between the behavior itself and the disorder stemming from that behavior [1]. A paraphilia by itself does not necessarily justify or require clinical intervention. In keeping with the distinction between paraphilias and paraphilic disorders, the term disorder should be reserved for individuals who meet both Criteria A (which specifies the qualitative nature of the paraphilia, e.g., an erotic focus on children or on exposing one's genitals to strangers) and B (which specifies the negative consequences of the paraphilia, i.e., distress, impairment, or harm to others). In addition, Criterion A delineates a signs and symptoms time span, indicating that they must persist for at least 6 months, to ensure that the atypical sexual interest is not merely transient [1].

DSM-5 describes eight specific disorders of this type, along with two residual categories called "paraphilias not otherwise specified" and "unspecific paraphilia disorder" (all listed in Table 2.1).

A.D. Fisher • M. Maggi (✉)
Sexual Medicine and Andrology Unit, Department of Experimental, Clinical and Biomedical Sciences, University of Florence, Viale Pieraccini 6, Florence 50139, Italy
e-mail: afisher@unifi.it; m.maggi@dfc.unifi.it

Table 2.1 Different kinds of paraphilias, according to the Diagnostic and Statistical Manual of Mental Disorders 5 Edition classification. Identification code numbers from DSM 5 are in parentheses

Voyeurism disorder (302.82)	Spying on an unsuspecting person who is naked/disrobed or engaged in sexual activity
Exhibitionism disorder (302.4)	Exposing one's genitals to unsuspecting persons (NOT the same as public urination)
Frotteurism disorder (302.89)	Touching and rubbing against a non-consenting person
Sexual masochism disorder (302.83)	Undergoing humiliation, bondage, or suffering
Sexual sadism disorder (302.84)	Inflicting humiliation, bondage, or suffering
Pedophilic disorder (302.2)	Sexually targeting children (perpetrator is ≥ 16 years old and ≥ 5 years older than the victim)
Fetishistic disorder (302.81)	Using nonliving objects as a repeatedly preferred or exclusive method of achieving sexual excitement (e.g., leather goods, clothing, undergarments, fabrics, shoes). (If female clothing is used in cross-dressing or devices are used to directly stimulate the genitals—e.g., vibrator—this is NOT a fetishism)
Transvestic fetishistic disorder (302.3)	Wearing clothing of the other sex for sexual arousal
Paraphilias not otherwise specified (302.9)	This category is included for coding paraphilias that do not meet the criteria for any of the specific categories. Examples include, but are not limited to, telephone scatologia (obscene phone calls), necrophilia (corpses), partialism (exclusive focus on a part of the body), zoophilia (animals), coprophilia (feces), klismaphilia (enemas), and urophilia (urine)
Unspecified paraphilic disorder (302.9)	Symptoms of paraphilic disorder that cause clinically significant distress or impairment in important areas of functioning but do not meet the full criteria for any of the disorders in the paraphilic disorders diagnostic class

2.1.2 Paraphilic Disorder and Sex Offenses

It is important to remember that not all sex offenders suffer from paraphilias, but only a part of them, and vice versa that not all patients with paraphilias are sex offenders [2]. In fact, often paraphilic individuals only suffer from deviant sexual fantasies or urges, or their deviant sexual behavior does not involve a non-consenting person or a child [2]. These individuals may present for treatment because of the associated distress in their personal lives.

In contrast, other paraphilic behaviors may lead to sex offenses, a major public health concern, defined as any violation of established legal or moral codes of sexual behavior. In fact, sex offending can cause a significant level of psychopathology, loss of quality of life and productivity, and an increase of mental health expenses in victims [3]. For example, clinically defined sexual behaviors such as pedophilia, voyeurism, frotteurism, and exhibitionism are considered sexual offenses but, for example, fetishism and transvestic fetishism are not.

On the other hand, crimes such as rape are not classified as paraphilias.

Simply having a paraphilia is clearly not illegal. Acting in response to paraphilic impulses, however, can be illegal [2].

2.1.3 Prevalence

Current prevalence figures are unavailable for all of the paraphilias. The prevalence of paraphilias is mainly derived from the prevalence of sex offenses. However, the latter is underestimated because many offenders have never been caught or the offense did not result in a conviction. In addition, many sexual assaults are undisclosed or unreported by the victim due to shame or feelings of guilt [4].

Recidivism is a major concern in the treatment of sex offenders with a paraphilic disorder, especially in pedophilia [2]. Published recidivism rates among pedophiles range from 10 % to 50 %, depending on how subjects are grouped. Incestuous (compared to non-related), homosexual, and bisexual (compared to heterosexual) pedophiles, as well as those with psychiatric comorbid disorders, addictive disorders (particularly alcoholism or drug abuse), or sociopathic or antisocial personality traits, exhibit higher rates of recidivism [5–7]. However, an instrument capable of predicting the future activity of a pedophilic individual does not exist.

2.2 Therapeutic Approaches

As incarceration alone has been reported by several authors as not solving sexual violence, treating the sexual offenders with a diagnosis of paraphilia is critical in an approach to preventing sexual violence and reducing victimization [2].

The heterogeneous characteristics of paraphilias request a comprehensive approach, in which different treatment options have to be integrative. In addition, treatment has to be individualized and adaptable to different client needs [6, 8–10]. The treatment modalities currently used in paraphiliac behaviors fall essentially into three categories:
1. Psychotherapy
2. Surgical castration
3. Pharmacotherapy

Whereas the goal of psychological interventions is to change the sexual behavior of the offender leaving the libido intact (and maintaining and enhancing normophilic sexual interests), pharmacological interventions seek to greatly reduce or completely eradicate sexual desire and capacity.

The aims of the treatment are to control paraphilic fantasies and behavior in order to decrease the risk of recidivism; to control sexual urges; and to decrease the level of distress of the paraphiliac subject.

2.2.1 Psychotherapy

Most commonly, psychotherapy is a combination of both individual and group-family therapy approaches [11]. Cognitive behavioral therapy (CBT) has been considered the non-pharmacologic "gold standard" approach which could be offered to pedophiles and its principles support most of the prison-based sex offender treatment programs [10, 12]. This type of approach consists in changing internal processes, together with changing overt behavior, such as social skills or coping behaviors. The goal of treatment is to decrease inappropriate sexual arousal and increase appropriate arousal [13].

In order to eliminate the pattern of sexual arousal to deviant stimuli, a variety of techniques can be used [14, 15]. Behavioral techniques to decrease sexual deviancy involve covert sensitization (imagining deviant sexual experience until arousal and then imagining an aversive experience), olfactory aversion conditioning (using an unpleasant smell, such as ammonia), aversion therapy (exposing client to deviant material followed by aversive stimulus), systemic desensitization (by paring relaxation with imagined scenes representing anxiety producing situations), and masturbatory satiation (making the deviant fantasy boring) [12].

The second component of CBT is to support the paraphilic individual in cultivating appropriate sexual response patterns. This could be obtained through several techniques, such as fading (fantasizing about atypical sexual stimuli and then gradually fading the fantasy into one concerning more acceptable sexual activity) or orgasmic reconditioning (in which the patient masturbates to orgasm while fantasizing about or watching normative sexual behavior) [12].

Moreover, treatments are designed to improve a sex offender's social competence, interpersonal and functional social skills, and self-esteem and to address intimacy deficits. The psychosocial treatment should include training in anger management, relaxation, and interventions to promote empathy with the victim and awareness. Irrational beliefs, such as beliefs that sex with children is a way to teach them about sexuality or that most women enjoy being raped, can contribute to an individual's justifying and engaging in deviant and criminal sexual behavior. Treatment to alter distorted beliefs involves the identification of and challenges to these kinds of cognitive distortions through cognitive restructuring techniques [12].

The evidence base for the efficacy of CBT for sex offenders is extremely limited, indicating only a modest reduction in recidivism and empirical research focusing on effective treatment for this population is needed critically [13–15]. Moreover, it should be considered that these kinds of approaches are costly. The other approaches (psychosocial programs, therapeutic communities, insight-orientated treatment) do not seem to reduce recidivism. In conclusion, currently there is still much debate regarding the overall effectiveness of psychotherapy approaches for the long-term prevention of new offenses and several studies have reported that the best outcomes in preventing repeat offenses against children occur when pharmacological agents and psychotherapy are combined together.

2.2.2 Surgical Castration

Orchidectomy apparently leads to definitive results, even in repeat pedophilic offenders, by reducing recidivism rates down to 2–5 % [16]. However, it is not always effective in producing impotence, as up to one-third of castrated males can still engage in sexual intercourse. From the introduction of surgical castration in 1892 in Switzerland (as a treatment for hypersexuality) until the 1970s, this procedure was used in many European countries and the United States. The substantial advantage of this procedure is linked to the difference in terms of cost between one-time surgical castration and ongoing "chemical castration" with pharmacological therapy, considering also limited prison healthcare budgets. This led to the state of Texas mandating the use of only surgical castration, the lone state among nine in the United States allowing surgical and/or "chemical castration."

On the other hand, since medication is available that produces similar results, the Belgian Advisory Committee on Bioethics [17] have recently advised that surgical castration no longer be an option for treatment of sex offenders.

2.2.3 Pharmacologic Treatments

Pharmacological therapies are used in order to reduce the general level of sexual arousal [18, 19].

2.2.3.1 Psychotropic Drugs

Lithium carbonate, tricyclic antidepressants (clomipramine, desimipramine), mirtazapine, antipsychotics (benperidol, thioridazine, haloperidol, risperidone), and anticovulsivants (carbamazepine, topiramate, divalproate) have been occasionally used over the years [8]. However, no randomized controlled trials have documented the efficacy of these psychotropic drugs in paraphilic sex offenders and the level of evidence is very poor.

Conversely, research evidence has demonstrated the efficacy of selective serotonin reuptake inhibitors (SSRIs) for treatment of paraphilic sexual offenders [20–22]. The rationale for the use of SSRIs in sexual offenders is based on various evidence [23, 24]:

- Increased levels of serotonin in the hypothalamus are able to inhibit sexual motivation and the testosterone signal.
- Higher levels of serotonin in the prefrontal cortex enhance emotional resilience and impulse control.
- SSRIs have been shown to decrease impulsiveness in antisocial impulsivity, anxiety, depression, and hypersexuality.
- Their use in treating Axis 1 and Axis 2 disorders, which are often comorbid with paraphilic disorders

The most studied SSRIs for the treatment of sex offenders with paraphilias are fluoxetine and sertraline. The preferred strategy is dose titration until a significant reduction or absence of symptoms is obtained [25].

2.2.3.2 Androgen Deprivation

Androgens play a crucial role in sexual interest and associated sexual arousability, which is defined as a state that motivates the individual toward the experience of sexual pleasure and possibly orgasm [26]. Therefore, a reduction in circulating testosterone levels results in decreasing sexual interest, arousability, fantasies, and behavior and may be consequently helpful in reducing or abolishing the paraphilic manifestations [26].

In addition, it has been reported that testosterone levels predict sexual recidivism and higher levels are associated with more invasive sexual crimes in sexual offenders. In fact, diminishing the intensity of the eroticized urges through androgen deprivation therapy may facilitate the resisting of those urges [8].

However, normal levels of testosterone play a crucial role in bone health, cardiovascular and metabolic systems, mood, erythropoiesis, sebaceous gland activities, and several other functions. Consequently, androgen deprivation leads to several pathological effects on these biological systems [21]. In particular, regarding bone health, androgen deprivation therapy induces bone mineral density decrease (typically in the spine, hip, and forearm, but also at appendicular skeletal sites such as the femoral neck). Bone loss usually occurs within 1 year after the start of androgen deprivation therapy, with a continuing reduction thereafter (approximately 3–7 % per year in lumbar spine). The resulting increased risk of osteoporotic fracture is also exacerbated by changes in body composition induced by hormonal castration, such as increases in weight and body mass index and reductions in lean body mass and muscle mass/strength. Hence, it is recommended that bone mineral density be measured by dual energy x-ray absorptiometry (DEXA) before starting androgen deprivation therapy (particularly in individuals at high risk), in order to detect preexisting osteoporosis and to monitor bone loss over time [21]. Effective prophylactic and therapeutic strategies for this musculoskeletal effect can include calcium (1,200–1,500 mg/day) and vitamin D supplementation (400–800 IU daily). Patients should be advised to abstain from smoking and excessive alcohol use. Moreover, bisphosphonate (e.g., oral alendronate or risedronate, and parental pamidronate or zoledronic) is recommended in men with preexisting osteopenia, osteoporosis, or fractures due to minimal trauma and has been successfully used in reducing bone loss in hormonally castrated patients. Moreover, parathyroid hormone (or a congener such as teriparatide) therapy and selective estrogen receptor modulators, such as raloxifene, are also being investigated. Finally, a low-dose androgen supplementation (e.g., testosterone enanthate 25–50 mg/month) has been considered. The latter may also improve erectile failure, enhancing an appropriate sexual relationship with partners, although all paraphilic manifestations usually remain totally suppressed [21].

Moreover, men treated with hormonal castration develop an increase in fat mass, hyperinsulinemia, hyperglycemia, insulin resistance, and impaired lipid profile, which lead to a higher risk of metabolic syndrome, diabetes mellitus (by 40–50 %), and cardiovascular diseases (by 10–20 %). To limit these side effects, it is important that patients adopt a healthy lifestyle and dietary behaviors, including smoking cessation and regular exercise. Statin therapy can be added if target levels are not reached (low-density lipoprotein cholesterol levels, <2.6 mmol/l or 100 mg/dl; fasting triglycerides levels, <1.7 mmol/l or 150 mg/dl; high-density lipoprotein cholesterol levels, >1.1 mmol/l or 40 mg/dl) by such non pharmacological interventions [21].

Concerning mood, low testosterone levels have been associated with an increased risk of depression, emotional disturbances, anxiety, fatigue, malaise, memory difficulties, asthenia, and apathy. In this regard, it should be further taken into account that paraphilic individuals suffer frequently from comorbid affective disorders or other mental illness. Moreover, conviction, imprisonment, and the stigma and shame of being a sexual offender may also increase the risk of depression after the start of hormonal deprivation therapy [8]. Therefore, sex offenders should be carefully evaluated before starting and during androgen deprivation therapy for the presence of mental illness, to provide appropriate psychiatric treatment.

Other side effects of hormonal therapy include hot flushes and night sweating, which may affect quality of life. Hot flushes can be effectively treated with SSRIs and selective serotonin–norepinephrine reuptake inhibitors, which also may be beneficial in treating comorbid depressive symptoms.

In addition, other side effects that have been described are breast tenderness and gynecomastia. Radiation (at a single dose of 1,500 cGy per breast) has been used to prevent or treat painful gynecomastia in these patients.

Furthermore, besides impotence and hypoactive sexual desire, androgen deprivation therapy also induces partial azospermia and infertility, although it does not provide birth control assurance.

Beyond the aforementioned side effects common to androgen deprivation agents, the single compound-specific side effects (e.g., hepatotoxicity for cyproterone acetate) listed in each dedicated paragraph should also be taken into account.

For all these reasons, effective and wise management of sex offenders treated with androgen deprivation therapy should include careful monitoring of side effects and their prevention with treatment. In addition, sex offenders who start treatment should be aware that this intervention is not without its risks.

2.2.3.2.1 Steroidal Antiandrogens

These compounds interfere with the binding of dihydrotestosterone (DHT, the androgen which plays the dominant role in androgenic response) to androgen receptors and they have been shown to block the cellular uptake of androgens. In addition, due to their powerful progestational activity, they cause inhibition of gonadotropin secretion and block their expected compensatory rise following a decrease in serum testosterone levels. Consequently, the inhibition of LH secretion results in a decrease of both testosterone and DHT levels. This latter effect is in contrast with that of the pure antiandrogens (e.g., flutamide). In fact, when pure antiandrogens compete with testosterone in binding to androgen receptors, a compensatory rise in gonadotropin secretion occurs; this increase, in turn, stimulates testosterone production and eventually overcomes receptor blockade.

Cyproterone Acetate

Cyproterone acetate (CPA) is a synthetic steroid, with three potential mechanisms underlying its antiandrogenic effects: (a) It inhibits the intracellular uptake and metabolism of androgens, blocking their binding to receptors (including brain ones), through competitive inhibitions; (b) it blocks testosterone (and estrogen) synthesis in the gonads; and (c) it has the progestational effect mentioned above [27, 28]. The antiandrogenic effect of CPA is believed to outweigh the progestational effect in terms of clinical efficacy in paraphilia treatment; however, it is the progestational effect that allows safe and effective long-term therapy. Equilibrium between these two influences requires many months of treatment (8–15 months on 100 mg/day and 15–20 months on 200 mg/day).

CPA has been approved for the treatment of the sex drive in sexual deviants in many countries and it is the most widely studied agent for the treatment of sex offenders with paraphilic disorders [8]. It can be prescribed in oral (usual regimen, 50–200 mg/day; maximum, 600 mg/day) or intramuscular (IM) depot formulations (200–400 mg once weekly or every 2 weeks) [8].

Apart from the aforementioned adverse effects related to hypogonadism, CPA-specific side effects include venous thromboembolism (VTE), adrenal insufficiency or hyperplasia, increased body weight, and local pain in the injection site (when IM formulations are used). Although large doses of CPA can produce hepatomas in rats, no evidence exists that the same happens in humans. Consequently, serious hepatotoxicity is not a common finding with CPA (less than 1 %). A history of VTE or recent surgery or trauma increases the risk of thromboembolic phenomena (by 4- and 13-fold, respectively).

Compared with the oral formulation, injectable CPA (via IM depot injection) shows a lower tolerability, in terms of local pain (at the injection site), joint/muscle pain, headache, sleep disturbances, and nausea.

Before treatment with CPA, evaluating and addressing conditions that can be exacerbated by this treatment are recommended, as is checking testosterone, FSH, LH, and prolactin plasma levels, liver function, blood cell count, electrocardiogram, fasting glucose blood level, blood pressure, weight, calcium and phosphate blood levels, kidney function, and bone mineral density.

During CPA treatment, biochemical monitoring of liver function must be evaluated every month for 3 months and then every 3–6 months; prolactin, glucose blood levels, blood cell count, calcium and phosphate blood levels, blood pressure, and weight every 6 months; and bone mineral density once a year (particularly, in the case of increased osteoporosis risk).

In addition, patients have to be evaluated every 1–2 months for emotional disturbances and depression by a mental health professional.

Regarding the efficacy of CPA in paraphilic sex offenders, studies reported a decrease of referred sexual fantasies and activities in 80–90 % of subjects, with a rate of re-offending of 6 % (vs 85 % in those without treatment). The majority of re-offenders were those who did not properly adhere to treatment prescription [29].

Medroxyprogesterone Acetate

Compared to CPA, medroxyprogesterone acetate (MPA) is less potent as an antiandrogen and progestogen and relatively more progestogenic than antiandrogenic (as opposed to the "balanced" effects with cyproterone acetate). A complete ablation of the testosterone levels is reached usually within 1–2 weeks after starting therapy. Moreover, MPA also induces the testosterone-α-reductase, which accelerates testosterone metabolism, and reduces plasma testosterone by enhancing its clearance.

MPA is available as oral tablets (usual regimen 100–400 mg/day) and parenteral suspensions for IM injections (usual regimen starts with 300 mg given weekly and then is titrated to achieve prepubertal testosterone levels) [30]. Erratic oral bioavailability (within and between products and within and between subjects) has made the IM formulation preferable and the majority of clinical trial data regarding MPA's use in abnormal sexual behaviors has been generated using the IM formulation.

Usually, reduction of sexual behavior and complete disappearance of deviant sexual behavior and fantasies is observed after 1–2 months of treatment.

Adverse events related specifically to MPA treatment included VTE, pulmonary embolism, excessive weight gain, headache, malaise, dyspepsia, muscle cramps, gallstones, diabetes mellitus, adrenal suppression, and Cushing syndrome [19, 31]. A recent study has reported the balanced effects on D-dimer levels and activated partial thromboplastin time values (which have opposing effects on VTE risk) in a sample of women using MPA. This latter result suggests that the potential risk of VTE with MPA may be lower than once thought.

MPA was the first drug studied in the treatment of paraphilias. Unfortunately, most studies were not controlled and some biases were observed. Moreover, considering the severe side effects observed with MPA, the benefit/risk ratio seems not to be favorable and, therefore, its use has been limited [2].

In any case, if clinicians decide to initiate MPA therapy for a paraphilia, they have to take its toxicity potential into consideration and, in an attempt to prevent or ameliorate adverse events, the dose may be lowered, at the cost of reduced therapeutic efficacy. The use of MPA has to be carefully managed medically, via physical examination, especially for the effects of feminization.

The schedule for clinical assessment of individuals treated with MPA is the same as has been suggested for CPA treatment.

2.2.3.2.2 Long-Acting Analogues of Gonadotropin-Releasing Hormone

Long-Acting Analogues of Gonadotropin-Releasing Hormone Agonists (GnRHa) are approved in many countries for a variety of pediatric, obstetric and gynecological, and oncological disorders, such as central precocious puberty, endometriosis, uterine fibromyomas, breast cancer (in premenopausal women), and advanced prostate cancer. Recently, they have also been used in adolescents with Gender Dysphoria [32].

GnRHa produce a complete chemical castration with hypoandrogenism as the only clinical effect. Although during the first weeks of treatment the release of LH and FSH is stimulated, leading to elevations in sex hormone blood concentrations ("flare-up"), continued use results in a suppression on account of the depletion and desensitizing of the gonadotrope hypophyse cells. The result is reduced LH and FSH secretion and thus reduced sex hormone production until castrated levels are reached, within 2–4 weeks. Because the initial rise of testosterone is theoretically associated with increased deviant sexual arousal or behavior, concurrent use of a pure antiandrogen (CPA or flutamide) is recommended during the initial weeks of GnRHa use.

In addition, GnRH containing neurons project into pituitary and extrapituitary sites, such as the olfactory bulb or the amygdala. At these latter sites, GnRH is believed to act as a neuromodulator and, through this action, may also be involved in sexual behavior. Thus, GnRHa, by inducing castrate testosterone levels, progressively lead to and maintain the inhibition of the fundamental elements of male sexuality: sexual fantasies, desire, and interest in sexual activities, resulting in either a dramatic decrease or an abolishment of the sexually deviant behavior [24].

Three analogues of the gonadotropin-releasing hormone are available.

Triptorelin is a synthetic decapetptide agonist, recently approved in Europe for the reversible decrease in plasma testosterone to castration levels in order to reduce drive in sexual deviations of adult men. It was developed as a monthly or depot formulation (3 mg, 1-month formulation or 11.25 mg, 3-month formulation) [33–36].

Leuprolide is a synthetic GnRHa, developed as daily IM or depot injections (3.75 or 7 mg, 1-month or 22.5 mg, 3-month formulation) [37, 38].

Gasorelin is also a synthetic GnRHa, developed as daily IM or depot injections (3.6 mg or 10.8 mg, subcutaneously) [39, 40].

No studies have compared the efficacy of these three medications [8].

Apart from the general adverse effects linked to androgen deprivation reported above and possible injection-site reactions (induration, burning, redness, itching, bruising, and pain), GnRHa appear to be a safe treatment.

Despite there not being any randomized controlled studies and some biases having been observed in open trials conducted with GnRHa, in the majority of cases these drugs have shown a better efficacy when compared to psychotherapy, SSRIs, or other antiandrogens [8, 33–37, 39, 40]. In addition, GnRHa are associated with lower rates of side effects, if compared with CPA and MPA [39]. Finally, poor compliance is often associated with oral CPA treatment, whereas long-acting CPA may increase treatment adherence. On this basis, the World Federation of Societies of Biological Psychiatry (WFSBP) guidelines underline that GnRHa treatment probably constitutes the most promising treatment for sex offenders at high risk for sexual violence, such as pedophiles or serial rapists.

The schedule for clinical assessment of individuals treated with GnRHa is the same as has been suggested for CPA and MPA treatment.

In summary, the different medical options available for hormonal castrations are characterized by and differ in terms of:
- efficacy
    - MPA, CPA, or GnRHa significantly reduce the intensity and the frequency of sexual arousal, but do not change the content of paraphilias;

- GnRHa are more potent than CPA or MPA in reducing testosterone levels more dramatically and more consistently;
- side effects
  - MPA and CPA are associated with a high percentage of side effects which have considerably limited their use;
  - GnRHa induce fewer side effects (except for those related to hypoandrogenism);
- patient's compliance
  - uncontrolled breaks in the therapy are often observed with CPA or MPA treatments;
  - GnRHa may be administered parenterally once every 1–3 months, producing less variable results in the treatment of paraphiliac behavior than CPA and MPA.

Algorithm of Treatment of Paraphilias

A treatment program should start with supportive psychotherapy and, in most cases, CBT. In all cases, treatment of comorbidities is necessary if any are present (Level 1). In the presence of psychiatric comorbidities, pharmacological treatment such as benzodiazepines, antipsychotics, SSRIs, or specific types of psychotherapies must be used.

In mild cases with strong deviant fantasies or impulses and any risk of sexual offenses, psychotherapy in combination with SSRI treatment should be considered, especially if the paraphilic patient shows additional symptoms such as anxiety, social phobia, depression, severe feelings of guilt, obsession, or personality disorders and if paraphilia is less severe (Level 2).

If there is insufficient improvement and a moderate-to-high risk of "hands-on" offenses, low doses of antiandrogens, preferentially in combination with SSRIs, should be given. Side effects are dose related, so a careful titration could minimize them and may allow patients to maintain appropriate sexual behavior while eliminating deviant behavior (Level 3).

Full dosage of CPA (or, if not available, MPA) should be added to SSRI treatment in subjects with moderate and high risk of sexual offense (severe paraphilias with more intrusive fondling with a limited number of victims), considering the intramuscular application in not compliant patients (Level 4).

In high risk of sexual offenses and severe paraphilias, sexual sadism fantasies and/or behavior or physical violence, and no compliance or no satisfactory results at Level 4, use of GnRH agonist could be justifiable and helpful (Level 5).

Finally, in the most severe paraphilias, a combination of antiandrogens, GnRH agonist, and SSRI must be considered (Level 6).

In case of serious side effects (VTE or severe liver dysfunction) CPA or MPA treatment must be replaced with GnRHa.

For a summary of the treatment algorithm, see also Fig. 2.1.

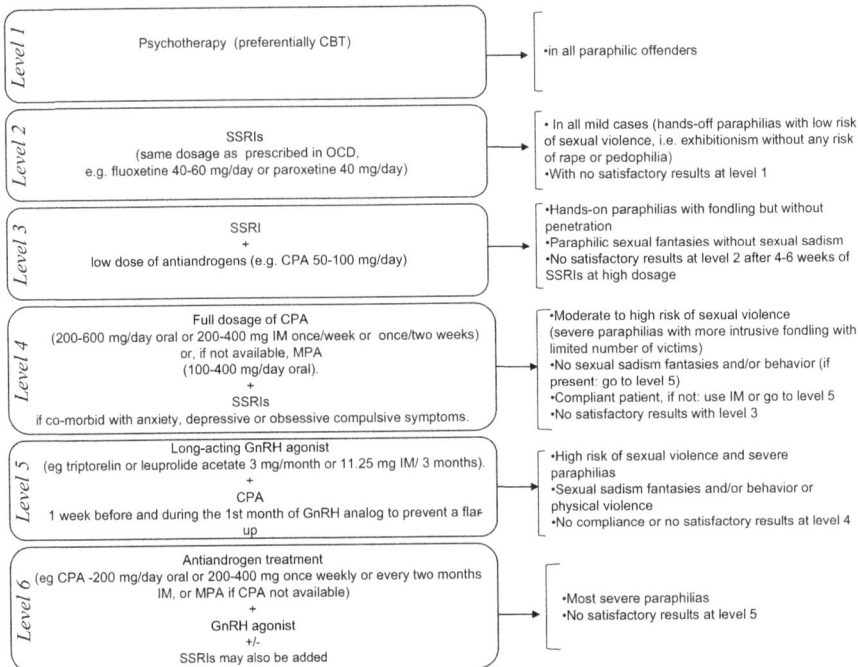

Fig. 2.1 Treatment algorithm of paraphilias, modified from Thibaut F, et al The World Federation of Societies of Biological Psychiatry (WFSBP) Guidelines for the biological treatment of paraphilias. *The Journal of Biological Psychiatry, 2010;11:604–655. CBT* cognitive behavioral therapy, *OCD* obsessive–compulsive disorder

Treatment Duration

Paraphilia is a chronic disorder and sexual orientation will not change during treatment.

For severe paraphilia with a high risk of sexual violence a minimal duration of treatment of 3–5 years is necessary. In these patients in particular, hormonal treatment must not be abruptly stopped [2].

Ethical Issues

The treatment of paraphilic sex offenders, irrespective of which method of treatment is employed, has always been undertaken with clinical and ethical dilemmas [9].

The major ethical issues may reflect the dispute between the need for public safety and, on the other side, the consent of the patient to be treated. Moreover, such kinds of crimes bring the public and even professional orientation toward punishment rather than treatment, even if appropriate and effective. For example, incarceration may stop pedophiles from committing illegal sexual acts against children, but it does not change the pedophile's internal sexual preference [9].

In some countries, paraphilic sex offenders may be ordered by the judge to undergo treatment as part of the rehabilitative aspect of sentencing, but these situations should leave treatment options up to professionals. Moreover, this decision should be made by a mental health professional with the requisite competence, after examination of the person concerned and after an informed consent has been obtained. However, doubts about the validity of consent have arisen, because consent is sometimes given in situations where the person is subject to some external pressure [9].

According to the European Ethics Board [17] if the paraphilic sex offenders need hormonal therapy, this should be allowed only if all of the following conditions are met:

- The person has a paraphiliac disorder diagnosed by a psychiatrist after a careful psychiatric examination.
- The hormonal treatment addresses specific clinical signs, symptoms, and behaviors and is adapted to the person's state of health. The hormonal treatment cannot be the only measure imposed on sex offenders on the basis of the nature of the crimes committed, but it must be integrated with a wider treatment program which also includes psychological and social aspects.
- The person's condition represents a significant risk of serious harm to his health or to the physical or moral integrity of other persons.
- The advice of an endocrinologist is mandatory when hormonal castration is considered.
- The hormonal treatment is a medical treatment for which the psychiatrist in charge of the patient takes responsibility (a) for the indication, (b) to inform the person involved and to receive his consent (c) for the follow-up, including somatic aspects with the help of a consulting endocrinologist, if necessary.
- The therapist will always give preference to the least intrusive intervention to obtain a particular result. If a less intrusive alternative treatment exists instead of hormonal treatment, this alternative must be preferred.
- The hormonal treatment is part of a written treatment plan to be reviewed at appropriate intervals and, if necessary, revised.

References

1. American Psychiatric Association. 2013. Diagnostic and statistical manual of mental disorders, 5th edn: DSM-5 tm. American Psychiatric Association, Washington, DC
2. Thibaut F (2012) Pharmacological treatment of paraphilias. Isr J Psychiatry Relat Sci 49: 297–305
3. Post L, Mezey N, Maxwell N, Wilbert W (2002) The rape tax: tangible and intangible costs of sexual violence. J Interpers Violence 17:773–782
4. Birger M, Bergman-Levy T, Asman O (2011) Treatment of sex offenders in Israeli prison settings. J Am Acad Psychiatry Law 39:100–103
5. Craig LA, Browne KD, Stringer I, Hogue TE (2008) Sexual reconviction rates in the United Kingdom and actuarial risk estimates. Child Abuse Negl 32:121–138
6. Hanson RK, Morton KE, Harris AJ (2003) Sexual offender recidivism risk: what we know and what we need to know. Ann NY Acad Sci 989:154–166

7. Hanson RK, Morton-Bourgon KE (2005) The characteristics of persistent sexual offenders: a meta-analysis of recidivism studies. J Consult Clin Psychol 73:1154–1163
8. Garcia FD, Delavenne HG, Assumpção AF, Thibaut F (2013) Pharmacologic treatment of sex offenders with paraphilic disorder. Curr Psychiatry Rep 15:356
9. Thibaut F, De la Barra F, Gordon H, Cosyns P, Bradford JM, WFSBP Task Force on Sexual Disorders (2010) The World Federation of Society of biological Psychiatry (WFSBP) Guidelines for the biological treatment of paraphilias. J Biol Psychiatry 11:604–655
10. Hall RC (2007) A profile of pedophilia: definition, characteristics of offenders, recidivism, treatment outcomes, and forensic issues. Mayo Clin Proc 82:457–471
11. Kenworthy T, Adams CE, Bilby C, Brooks-Gordon B, Fenton M (2008) WITHDRAWN: psychological interventions for those who have sexually offended or are at risk of offending. Cochrane Database Syst Rev 4, CD004858
12. Kaplan MS, Krueger RB (2012) Cognitive-behavioral treatment of the paraphilias. Isr J Psychiatry Relat Sci 49:291–296
13. Losel F, Schmucker M (2005) The effectiveness of treatment for sexual offenders: a comprehensive meta-analysis. J Exp Criminol 1:117–146
14. Kenworthy T, Adams CE, Bilby C, Brooks-Gordon B, Fenton M (2004) Psychological interventions for those who have sexually offended or are at risk of offending. Cochrane Database Syst Rev 3:CD004858
15. Maletzki BM, Steinhauser C (2002) A 25-year follow-up of cognitive-behavioural therapy with 7,275 sexual offenders. Behav Modif 26:123–147
16. Brooks-Gordon B, Bilby C, Wells H (2006) A systematic review of psychological interventions for sexual offenders I. Randomised control trials. J Forensic Psychiatry 17: 442–466
17. Belgian Advisory Commitee on Bioethics (2006) Opinion no. 39 of December 18th 2006 on hormonal treatment of sex offender. http://www.health.belgium.be/internet2Prd/groups/public/@public/@dg1/@legalmanagement/documents/ie2divers/18074794.pdf. Accessed 25 Jan 2014
18. Khan O, Ferriter M, Huband N, Smailagic N (2009) Pharmacological interventions for those who have sexually offended or are at risk of offending (Protocol). The Cochrane Library, Issue 3
19. Guay DRP (2009) Drug treatment of paraphilic and nonparaphilic sexual disorders. Clin Ther 31:1–31
20. Adi Y, Ashcroft D, Browne K, Beech A, Fry-Smith A, Hyde C (2002) Clinical effectiveness and cost-consequences of selective serotonin reuptake inhibitors in the treatment of sex offenders. Health Technol Assess 6:1–66
21. Thibaut F (2011) Pharmacological treatment of sex offenders. Sexologies 20:166–168
22. Fedoroff JP (1995) Antiandrogens vs serotonergic medications in the treatment of sex offenders: a preliminary compliance study. Can J Hum Sex 4:111–123
23. Meston CM, Frohlich PF (2000) The neurobiology of sexual function. Arch Gen Psychiatry 57:1012–1030
24. Hill A, Briken P, Kraus C, Strohm K, Berner W (2003) Differential pharmacological treatment of paraphilias and sex offenders. Int J Offender Ther Comp Criminol 47:407–421
25. Garcia FD, Thibaut F (2011) Current concepts in the pharmacotherapy of paraphilias. Drugs 71:771–790
26. Giltay EJ, Gooren LG (2009) Potential side effects of androgen deprivation treatment in sex offenders. J Am Acad Psychiatry Law 37:53–58
27. Jeffcoate WJ, Matthews RW, Edwards CR, Field LH, Besser GM (1980) The effect of cyproterone acetate on serum testosterone, LH, FSH and prolactin in male sexual offenders. Clin Endocrinol 13:189–195
28. Neuman F (1997) Pharmacology and potential use of cyproterone acetate. Horm Metab Res 9: 1–13

29. Dunsieth NW, Nelson EB, Brusman-Lovins LA, Holcomb JL, Beckman D, Welge JA et al (2004) Psychiatric and legal features of 113 men convicted of sexual offenses. J Clin Psychiatry 65:293–300
30. Bradford JM (2001) The neurobiology, neuropharmacology, and pharmacological treatment of the paraphilias and compulsive sexual behaviour. Can J Psychiatry 6:26–34
31. Raymons NC, Coleman E, Ohlerking F, Christenson GA, Miner M (1999) Psychiatric co-morbidity in pedophilic sex offenders. Am J Psychiatry 156:786–788
32. Hembree WC, Cohen-Kettenis P, Delemarre-van de Waal HA, Gooren LJ, Meyer WJ III, Spack NP, Tangpricha V, Montori VM (2009) Endocrine Society. Endocrine treatment of transsexuals persons: an Endocrine Society clinical practice guideline. J Clin Endocrinol Metab 94:3132–3154
33. Rosler A, Witztum E (2000) Pharmacotherapy of paraphilias in the next millennium. Behav Sci Law Behav Sci 18:43–56
34. Thibaut F, Cordier B, Kuhn JM (1993) Effect of a long-lasting gonadotrophin hormone-releasing hormone agonist in six cases of severe male paraphilia. Acta Psychiatr Scand 87: 445–450
35. Thibaut F, Cordier B, Kuhn JM (1996) Gonadotropin hormone releasing hormone agonist in cases of severe paraphilia: a lifetime treatment? Psychoneuroendocrinology 21:411–419
36. Thibaut F, Kuhn JM, Cordier B, Petit M (1998) Hormone treatment of sex offenses. Encéphale 24:132–137
37. Schober JM, Kuhn PJ, Kovacs PG, Earle JH, Byrne PM, Fries RA (2005) Leuprolide acetate suppresses pedophilic urges and arousability. Arch Sex Behav 34:691–705
38. Krueger RB, Kaplan MS (2001) Depot-Leuprolide Acetate for treatment of paraphilias: a report of twelve cases. Arch Sex Behav 30:409–422
39. Czerny JP, Briken P, Berner W (2002) Antihormonal treatment of paraphilic patients in German forensic psychiatric clinics. Eur Psychiatry 17:104–106
40. Brahams D (1988) Voluntary chemical castration of a mental patient. Lancet 1:1291–1292

Negative Attitudes to Lesbians and Gay Men: Persecutors and Victims

Vittorio Lingiardi and Nicola Nardelli

3.1 Homophobia Has Many Names

Homophobia, heterosexism, homonegativity, and sexual prejudice are all terms that are used to refer to negative attitudes towards homosexuality, lesbians, and gay men, but the most widely used is "homophobia." It was coined by George Weinberg in 1972 [1], who focused on the emotional components of the prejudice rather than cognitive ones. The important role Weinberg played in shifting the focus of scientific research from homosexuality to antigay hostility must be acknowledged, but our thinking on this concept [2] should be updated. The Greek suffix "phobia" means that the term implies unpleasant physiological and psychological reactions in the presence of gay people and the criteria for a clinical diagnosis of "phobia" include an excessive, irrational, inappropriate, and persistent fear of an object or circumstance, and the consequent desire to distance oneself from it. These criteria are not always and not necessarily satisfied by the concept of homophobia as commonly recognized, because (a) people with antigay attitudes consider their negative reactions towards lesbians and gay men to be normal and justifiable; (b) unlike phobias in the strict sense, homophobia does not necessarily compromise the social functioning of people with antigay attitudes; (c) homophobic people do not experience distress nor feel the need to get rid of negative attitudes; (d) phobias entail avoidance of feared objects or situations, while in homophobia avoidance behaviors can coexist with behaviors characterized by active aversion or deliberate aggression (for further reasons for abolishing the term "homophobia," see [2]).

The term "homophobia" is therefore not wholly appropriate as it focuses primarily on individual cases, neglecting the cultural component and the social roots of intolerance and hence the relationship between "homophobia" and other forms of "hating in the first person plural" (e.g., misogyny, racism, anti-Semitism, etc. [3]).

V. Lingiardi (✉) • N. Nardelli
Department of Dynamic and Clinical Psychology, Sapienza University of Rome, Via degli Apuli 1, Roma 00185, Italy
e-mail: vittorio.lingiardi@uniroma1.it; nicola.nardelli@uniroma1.it

Like racists and anti-Semites, antigay people usually refer to a codified system of beliefs framed in terms of the need to guard against people and values considered to be dangerous.

Negative attitudes towards homosexuality are rooted in primitive human anxieties about extinction and gender subversions, the latter first identified by Freud [4], that evoke the twin bogeys of male "passivity" and female "activity." As often happens, fear is transformed into hatred towards that which is perceived as different, whether it is external or internal to the self. A woman who loves another woman overturns the patriarchal rule that a woman is "completed" only by a penis that penetrates and fertilizes her. A man who loves another man gives up his "patriarchal vocation" and evokes the ghost of the penetration, then the passivity, then the feminization. The very 'gaze of a homosexual male is seen as contaminating,' writes the philosopher Martha Nussbaum [5, p. 114], 'because it says "You can be penetrated".'

Homophobia could also result from an individual's own conflicted homosexual feelings. As Freud [6] pointed out, using reactive formation and projection as defense mechanisms, conflicts related to unacceptable impulses can be transformed into hatred of objects representing them and to that extent may generate paranoia. Adams, Wright, and Lohr [7] provided further empirical evidence supportive of psychodynamic theories and their connection with cognitive science using a well-known paradigm also reported on by Westen [8]. A sample consisting of 64 exclusively heterosexual men was divided into two groups using the Index of Homophobia [9]. Both groups were exposed to sexually explicit erotic stimuli—consisting of heterosexual, gay male, and lesbian videotapes—while changes in penile circumference were monitored as a measure of arousal. Both groups showed increased arousal in association with heterosexual and lesbian erotic stimuli, whereas only participants within the "homophobic group" showed a penile erection increment in association with gay male erotic stimuli (for further reference to antigay hostility as a defense mechanism see [10]; for other empirical studies see [11]).

Negative attitudes toward homosexuality are pervasive in individuals and societal systems; it is important to understand each level where they occur: (1) individual level; (2) interpersonal level; (3) institutional level; and (4) cultural or societal level [12, 13].

Expressions of homosexuality—and homophobia—change with time and culture, from generation to generation. Some authors have considered it useful to distinguish between an old-fashioned form of prejudice and a modern one [14–16]. Morrison and Morrison [15], for example, argued that students' antigay prejudice shifted from moral and religious objections to homosexuality to more abstract concerns such as believing that lesbians and gay men were making illegitimate or unnecessary demands for social change (e.g., claims for spousal benefits).

Herek, Gillis, and Cogan [17] set out a social psychological framework that distinguished between the societal and institutional manifestations of homosexual stigma (heterosexism) and individual manifestations of internalized sexual stigma (specifically, sexual prejudice refers to negative attitudes toward homosexuality and sexual minorities, while self-stigma refers to negative attitudes toward oneself as homosexual or bisexual). Having provided a summary of the various forms of homonegativity and sexual prejudice, from the most explicit and violent ("gay bashing") to the most implicit and subtle, even supposedly "tolerant," we will turn to the issues of whether and how homonegativity might be measured.

3.2 Evaluating Sexual Prejudice and Self-Stigma

There are many instruments used to measure homonegativity. Most are self-report questionnaires. However, given that self-report measures detect primarily what the subject knows and is willing to state about him- or herself and considering the likely social desirability bias, such questionnaires will not capture antigay prejudice at the implicit level of awareness or prejudice masked by a desire to appear socially acceptable.

Implicit antigay attitudes have been studied by the *Implicit Association Test* (IAT) [18], which was shown to be a reliable measure in this domain [19]. The IAT assumes that automatic attitudes influence thoughts, feelings, and behaviors and therefore uses a computer-assisted categorization task to evaluate implicit attitudes through priming procedures. The test measures the latency of automatic associations between symbols representing a group (e.g., pictures of gay couples and pictures of heterosexual couples) and positive and negative words (e.g., good and bad). It assumes that antigay people more quickly associate pictures of lesbian or gay couples with negative words and pictures of heterosexual couples with positive words (and vice versa). The IAT compares two different categories, but sometimes it is necessary to test attitudes toward a single category. The Single Category IAT (SC-IAT) [20] was developed to meet this need. The IAT and SC-IAT have proved useful for attitude detection in a domain in which explicit attitudes may be significantly distorted by impression management; it has been shown that whilst heterosexual people showed positive explicit attitudes toward gays, implicit attitudes were relatively negative [21].

Nevertheless, self-report questionnaires are more versatile and easier to use, especially in large sample studies. Just as there are many terms to describe antigay attitudes, there are different constructions of antigay prejudice, each entailing differences in etiology, expression, and measurement [22, 23]. Some scales are one-dimensional and provide a single factor score, but there also multidimensional scales that provide multifactor scores. Given the association between gender and antigay prejudice, it may be important to recognize gender in assessment procedures. For example, the *Modern Homophobia Scale* (MHS) [16] (for an Italian study with the MHS, see [24]) assesses three dimensions of homophobia directed at lesbians and gay men: (a) *deviance*, the degree to which the respondent views homosexuality as deviant, pathological, and changeable; (b) *personal discomfort*, the urge to avoid personal contact with gay men and lesbians due to discomfort felt in their presence; and (c) *institutional homophobia*, opposition to recognizing the civil rights of lesbians and gay men.

There are also many instruments that assess self-stigma in lesbians and gay men. Exposed to social and institutional discrimination, gay and lesbian people may internalize prejudice, developing a distressing inner conflict that often has dramatic effects on self-esteem, psychological well-being, emotional state, and the quality of social and romantic relationships (this issue will be examined in depth in Sect. 3.4). Our *Measure of Internalized Sexual Stigma for Lesbians and Gay Men* (MISS-LG) [25] is available in two different forms—MISS-L for lesbians and MISS-G for gay men—it comprises 6 items dealing with gender-specific aspects and 11 items common to both forms (giving a total of 17 items in both forms). The scale assesses sexual stigma in lesbians and gay men in terms of three factors: (a) *identity*: the propensity to have a negative attitude to one's own homosexuality and consider sexual stigma as a part of a value system and identity; (b) *social discomfort*: fear of public identification as a lesbian or gay man in a social context; fear of disclosure in private and professional life and negative internalized beliefs about the religious, moral, and political acceptability of homosexuality; and (c) *sexuality*: a pessimistic evaluation of the quality or duration of gay or lesbian intimate relationships and a negative conception of gay or lesbian sexual behaviors.

3.3 Correlates of Antigay Prejudice

Often antigay prejudice works below the level of awareness. Operating the level of automatic and emotionally driven behavior, it appears to be stronger in people who are more sensitive to disgust. Disgust is a core emotion that has concrete, nonsocial, adaptive functions including facilitating the rejection of toxic or contaminated food and avoidance of disease [26]. However it may also manifest as a social, culturally adapted, broad-based emotion that motivates out-group avoidance [27] and mediates, for example, attitudes toward immigrants and foreigners [28]. Low status minorities often seem to elicit disgust [29] and recent research suggested that disgust may be implicated in antigay attitudes [30, 31]. Evolutionary psychology theories provide a clue to the possible role of disgust in the stigmatization of sexual behaviors [32]. These theories posit that disgust has developed from its origin as a disease-avoidance mechanism into a putative behavioral immune system consisting of a set of cognitive, affective, and behavioral tendencies to avoid sources of diseases. Because the biological costs of an infection are tremendously high, it makes evolutionary sense that a behavioral immune system would make a species hypervigilant and react to "false positive" threats. Thus a behavioral immune system could be triggered by people who appear "strange" to the societal majority because they do not conform to norms relating to food preparation, hygiene or sexual practices [30].

At the same time, several studies have emphasized that contact with gay people reduces sexual prejudice [33–35], suggesting that education is the key to the eradication of stereotypes and the reduction of prejudice and antigay hostility (for details on stereotypes and the influence of contact on prejudice, see [36]).

There are other important correlates of the sexual prejudice that we will examine briefly. First of all, religious fundamentalism and political conservatism are often associated with heterosexism, especially regarding civil rights, same-sex marriage, and parenting by lesbians and gay men [37, 38]. Gender is another important variable involved in antigay prejudice. In general, women seem less homophobic than men, and attitudes toward lesbians differ from attitudes toward gay men [10, 39–42]. In particular, it seems that antigay hostility is related to heightened levels of masculinity and is stronger in men who feel threatened by individuals perceived as "too feminine" [43]. Older people often have more negative attitudes toward sexual minorities than younger people (e.g., [39, 44]). Young people grew up in a social environment characterized by increasing respect for sexual minorities and are more likely have contact with publically identifying lesbian and gay men. Personality factors also show correlations with antigay prejudice, for example, "openness to experience" seems to be one of the best predictors of low sexual prejudice [33, 45, 46].

3.4 Minority Stress and Internalized Prejudice in Lesbians, Gay Men and Bisexuals

In 1973 the American Psychiatric Association (APA) removed the diagnosis of "ego-syntonic homosexuality" from the third edition of the Diagnostic and Statistical Manual of Mental Disorders (DSM-III). In 1987 the diagnosis of "ego-dystonic homosexuality" (undesired and conflicted homosexuality) was also removed. With these removals the APA recognized the link between heterosexism and internalized stigma in homosexual people. Lesbians, gay men, bisexuals, and all people with a nonheterosexual orientation, as well as transgender people (for convenience they are collectively conventionally referred to by the acronym LGBT), still risk harassment and other stressful and traumatic experiences. The incidence of distress and post-traumatic disorders is therefore significantly higher in sexual minorities than in heterosexual people [47–50]. At the same time, some studies have reported that the incidence of psychological distress and alcohol abuse among lesbians and gay men is significantly higher in countries without same-sex marriage laws, or more in generally without policies that protect sexual minorities against discrimination and violence [51–53], and in communities with an unsupportive religious climate [54].

Lesbians, gay men, and bisexuals are subjected to "minority stress." Unlike other minorities, they cannot always rely on the recognition and support of their family; in fact sometimes the converse: family may be an additional source of discomfort and stress. It is not unusual for homonegative dynamics to occur in a sociocultural context that is indifferent or even collusive. Episodes of discrimination and violence can have a very strong emotional impact that transcends their direct effects; they may affect not only direct victims, but also those who cannot avoid thinking that it might happen to them too.

Many studies of minority stress have confirmed its causal role in distress in lesbians and gay men (e.g., [50, 55–57]; for a review see [58]). Ilan Meyer [59]

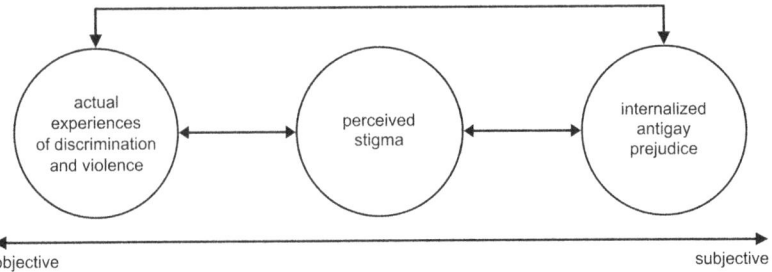

Fig. 3.1 The three dimensions of minority stress and the interactions among them, from the more objective to the more subjective

developed and tested a minority stress model in a community sample of 741 gay men. Odds ratios suggested that men who had high levels of minority stress were twice to three times more likely to suffer from high levels of distress as well. Meyer [60] suggested a distinction between distal and proximal causes of minority stress. This distinction relied on a conceptualization of stress that seems most relevant to minority stress. He described a minority stress continuum ranging from distal stressors—objective events and conditions—to proximal personal processes based on individual perceptions and appraisals. We can therefore construct a minority stress continuum extending from objective to subjective experiences that includes three dimensions: (a) *actual experiences of discrimination and violence*; (b) *perceived stigma*, i.e., expectations of rejection and discrimination; and (c) *internalized antigay prejudice*, direction of societal negative attitudes toward the self (Fig. 3.1).

The *internalized antigay prejudice* (also named internalized homophobia, internalized homonegativity, self-stigma, etc.) dimension is the set of negative feelings and attitudes (from discomfort to contempt) that a nonheterosexual person could experience (with various degrees of awareness) regarding her/his own sexual orientation. This could result in low self-acceptance and low self-esteem to self-hatred and self-contempt. Negative feelings may manifest in various ways and to varying degrees, including perhaps feelings of uncertainty, shame, and inferiority; inability to communicate one's sexual orientation to others; and the feeling of being rejected and self-identification with derogatory stereotypes.

Perceived stigma reflects vigilance and the fear of being "labeled" as lesbian or gay. The greater the perception of social rejection, the higher the degree of vigilance and sensitivity to the environment. Consequently, high levels of perceived stigma can lead to chronic stress and give rise to thoughts like "it only happened because I am homosexual," "I have to be careful not to say that I am gay or people will discriminate against me." Fear of the response to self-disclosure of sexual orientation to others—in the family as well as in the workplace—falls into this category.

3.5 The Impact of Minority Stress on Same-Sex Relationships

Minority stress may significantly affect the quality of relationships [61, 62, 99]. First of all, social prejudices and institutional discriminations jeopardize the well-being of same-sex couples. In addition to these obvious barriers lifelong discrimination, sexual stigma, and internalized prejudice are all consistently associated with lower relationship quality and partner abuse (e.g., [63–65]; for theoretical purposes, see also [66, 67]). The process by which lesbians and gay men acknowledge their homosexuality and come to feel comfortable being open about their identity is widely referred to as "coming out" (e.g., [68, 69]). Coming out plays an important role in relational life; therefore, it is necessary to pay attention to both the partner's and his or her own coming out.

Although there is still insufficient empirical research to draw general conclusions (for a methodological review see [70]), it is possible to identify two important aspects of domestic violence in same-sex couples.

The first aspect concerns silence about the abuse and the further social isolation of the victim. Internalized prejudice constitutes a considerable barrier to seeking help, as there is fear that one's sexual orientation will be perceived as justification for the abuse, as well as fear of antigay reactions from police officers, service providers, and even family members [71–74].

The second aspect concerns the potential negative affect of past stressful or traumatic experiences related to same-sex attraction. For example, antigay harassment might affect cognitive and psychological development resulting in an individual taking "revenge" on and seeking "compensation" from an intimate partner, thus undermining the intimacy of the relationship, as the following clinical vignette [62] illustrates:

> Antonio and Paolo have lived together for two years, but often they start fighting for pointless reasons and sometimes Antonio beats Paolo. At other times Antonio engages in sexually compulsive behaviors in which he penetrates and insults a hustler. He enters a state of fantasy-related hyperarousal in which he plays the role of a policeman raping a prisoner of war. It seems that Antonio's self-contempt, rage, and anxiety are enacted as dissociated and exciting fantasies that give him the opportunity to attribute these intolerable feelings to another person, and at the same time create the illusion of actively controlling them. Through the nonjudgmental listening, the psychiatrist gave Antonio the space he needed to focus on some aspects of his thoughts that he found unacceptable. Antonio's adolescence had been affected by feelings of shame and inferiority. He remembers having been bullied at school, something he has hardly ever spoken about, trying to forget it. He never disclosed his feelings to his parents, nor did he have the courage to tell them the stress he suffered as a result of being bullied at school. Furthermore, homosexuality has always been mocked and stigmatized by his family. In order to cope with these 'microaggressions of everyday life' [75], Antonio learned a dissociative defense mechanism, putting his identity as a 'faggot' in a sort of 'mental drawer', at the edge of his consciousness [66]. Every time he finds himself in a situation in which his homosexuality is detectable, it is as if episodic memories implicitly linked to his traumatic experience are reactivated. Even if he is not completely aware of it, Antonio expects that 'coming out' necessarily entails a negative reaction from somebody. On these occasions, feelings of anxiety, guilt and inferiority emerge, and Antonio tries to cope with them by identifying with the aggressor. In this way, he is 'turning the tables' and externalizing his distress. When problematic painful and

dissociated mental memories are reactivated (for example, when Paolo wants Antonio to introduce him to his parents), the burden of anxiety becomes too heavy and cannot be managed in a functional way anymore.

3.6 Homophobic Bullying

Homonegativity is displayed by young people inside and outside school walls. It is very pervasive and probably all children are exposed to its effects, which range from ridicule of gay people to disapproval and even violent attack. From childhood onwards both genders begin to experience negative stimuli related to homosexuality. Antigay bullying, often called homophobic bullying, is directed toward the victim's—actual or presumed—homosexual orientation or an atypical expression of gender which is contrary to sociocultural expectations. Students may be victimized because their parents or relatives are openly lesbian, gay, bisexual, or transgender. Like other common types of bullying, homophobic bullying can be divided into four main types of abuse: emotional, verbal, physical, and cyber-bullying.

It is widely recognized that victims of bullying are at risk of dropping out of school, developing stress-related, posttraumatic, or depressive disorders, and in extreme cases, suicide.

Compared to other forms of bullying, antigay bullying has several peculiarities: (a) the oppression concerns the nuclear identity dimensions of gender and sexuality and interferes with developmental processes which are already complicated by membership of a sexual minority; (b) the victim may experience particular difficulties in seeking help from adults because seeking help entails drawing attention to one's sexuality, which may be associated with feelings of anxiety and shame and a fear of disappointing expectations of heterosexuality and conformity with the norms of one's assigned gender; sometimes teachers and parents can act out homophobic prejudices, denying or underestimating the abuse, or worrying about the child's "abnormality" and looking for a "cure," or otherwise demonstrating rejection; (c) the victim may have particular trouble finding support and protection among peers because of the perceived risk of being considered gay; (d) antigay hostility may be part of a defensive internalized sexual prejudice, and through antigay behavior the bullies show that they are "normal guys" and affirm their conformity to gender expectations and give vent to any conflicting same-sex attraction or affect.

Another characteristic specific to antigay bullying concerns self-disclosure of sexual orientation. Observing the victimization of similar others may have a powerful effect, increasing fears and inhibiting young people from expressing themselves and thus jeopardizing their self-acceptance [76].

Mostly due to antigay bullying, young people who belong to a sexual minority or who question their own sexuality are less able to find social support than young people with more clearly defined identities; they report higher rates of victimization and show higher rates of school dropout, substance abuse, stress-related disorders, depressive symptoms, and suicide risk than heterosexual youths (e.g., [77, 78, 100]). Conversely a positive school climate can reduce differences in developmental outcomes.

The harmful of antigay bullying is not limited to mental health [79]. Research conducted by Holt, Matjasko, Espelage, Reid, and Koenig [80] provided confirmation of previous findings that bullying and sexual risk-taking behaviors were associated among adolescents: at the bivariate level, bullies and victims reported more casual sex and sex under the influence of alcohol and drugs than students who were not involved in bullying. Espelage, Basile, and Hamburger [81] also showed that there was a strong association between bullying and subsequent sexual harassment behavior, and between antigay teasing behaviors, co-occurring bullying behavior, and subsequent sexual harassment behavior. A meta-analysis by Marshal et al. [82] showed that on average 28 % of sexual minority young people reported a history of suicidal behavior compared with 12 % of heterosexual young people. Specific factors such as bisexuality or questioning one's sexuality and familial rejection were respectively associated with rates of suicidal behavior almost five times greater and eight times greater than in heterosexual young people [83]. Fortunately, many lesbian and gay young people have the ability and resources to cope successfully with traumatic experiences, reorganizing their lives positively and displaying resilience. The presence of a best friendship appears to be a protective factor [84].

The phenomenon of antigay bullying is clearly not negligible. United Nations Secretary-General Ban Ki-moon expressed deep concern about its global increase, stating that it constitutes a "grave violation of human rights" and that states were legally obliged to protect their citizens from this kind of violence: 'Tackling this problem is a shared challenge. We all have a role, whether as parents, family members, teachers, neighbours, community leaders, journalists, religious figures or public officials' (New York, 8 December 2011 [85]). The position of the United Nations was formalized in the *Rio Statement on Homophobic Bullying and Education for All* issued by UNESCO (Rio de Janeiro, 10 December 2011 [86]). The *Education for All* statement requires nation states to tackle threat anti-LGBT prejudice and violence pose to universal access to high-quality education by ensuring:

1. Safe schools and an educational climate free of anti-LGBTI prejudice and violence;
2. Access to accurate information on health and sexuality relevant to the needs of all learners, including LGBTI people;
3. Teachers and other school staff who are prepared and willing to maintain learning environments truly accessible and productive for all;
4. Mechanisms of periodic review by which educational institutions, systems, and governments consult with development partners and all education sector stakeholders in order to hold themselves accountable to the aforementioned principles.

Preventative policies and practices are indeed the best strategy against antigay bullying. They include appropriate educational spaces for staff and faculty, as well as appropriate psycho-educational interventions with students. Antigay bullying is most appropriately considered as a systemic problem, and preventative and care interventions should be targeted at entire classes rather than focusing solely on the victim and bully. Promoting an educational climate that is safe and welcoming for all students, including sexual minority and sexually questioning young people, is of fundamental importance. To achieve this inclusive curricula representing sexual minorities and their concerns and reducing their invisibility and marginalization are needed; this will also provide heterosexual young people with important learning opportunities. Resources for educators [87] are also needed. The *Gay, Lesbian, and Straight Education Network* website (GLSEN; http://www.glsen.org) includes a lot of useful resources.

3.7 Helping Victims Avoid Secondary Victimization

When victimization based on antigay prejudice occurs, the victim may conceal the event to avoid disclosure of his or her sexual orientation. The risk of further, secondary victimization is concrete: the victim knows this and may even anticipate it. Previous antigay experiences are associated with a learned anticipation of rejection and stigmatization by law enforcement agencies [88]. For sexual minorities secondary victimization carries specific risks: additional humiliation, loss of employment, eviction from housing, refusal of access to public accommodation, and loss of child custody [89]. Because secondary victimization is inflicted by those who should provide protection and support, secondary victimization may be even more distressing than the primary victimization. Victim-blaming is so a significant factor in determining well the victim copes with stressful and traumatic episodes [90].

Police officers, social service providers, educators, and legal and health practitioners should be careful not merely to avoid causing secondary victimization, but to create an environment in which the victim can feel secure and certain that he or she will not be stigmatized again. First, it is necessary to avoid displaying heteronormative bias by assuming that the victim is heterosexual (e.g., asking a girl if she has a boyfriend). Gay stereotypes (e.g., "you're like all gay men, too emotional") should also be avoided. Third, the victim's sexual orientation should not be used as a justification, in order to decriminalize the harassment (e.g., a teacher suggesting to a bullied child: "You should try to be less of a sissy").

Mental health professionals have to contemplate carefully the possibility that secondary victimization may have occurred in order to treat it as part of the traumatic event. It is important to avoid heterosexist and heteronormative bias. Although homosexuality is no longer considered a mental disorder by the scientific community [91], not all mental health professionals respect this in their practice; some continue to treat it as a mental disorder or a psychological impairment, making particular assumptions about its etiopathogenesis and providing interventions designed to alter sexual orientation [92, 93]. These interventions are often called "reparative therapies" because they are based on the biased assumption that homosexual orientation results from something that "went wrong" in personal development and therefore must be "repaired." The harmful consequences of efforts to alter sexual orientation are well recognized [94–97] (see Spitzer's letter to the editor of the *Archives of Sexual Behavior* reassessing his study supporting "reparative therapies" [98]). Sometimes adolescents are subjected to such interventions at their families' instigation and against their will. In other cases mental health professionals collude with clients' self-stigma. It should never be forgotten that providing these biased interventions is a violation of the first principle of medical ethics—*first, do no harm*—and is therefore a form of abuse.

References

1. Weinberg G (1972) Society and the healthy homosexual. St. Martin's Press, New York, NY
2. Herek GM (2004) Beyond "homophobia": thinking about sexual prejudice and stigma in the twenty-first century. Sex Res Social Policy 1(2):6–24
3. Moss D (ed) (2003) Hating in the first person plural: psychoanalytic essays on racism, homophobia, misogyny, and terror. Other Press, New York, NY
4. Freud S (11937) Analysis terminable and interminable. SE 23, pp 211–253
5. Nussbaum MC (2004) Hiding from humanity: disgust, shame and the law. Princeton University Press, Princeton, NJ
6. Freud S (1915–1917) Introductory lectures on psycho-analysis. SE 15–16
7. Adams HE, Wright LW Jr, Lohr BA (1996) Is homophobia associated with homosexual arousal? J Abnorm Psychol 105:440–445
8. Westen D (1998) The scientific legacy of Sigmund Freud: toward a psychodynamically informed psychological science. Psychol Bull 124:333–371
9. Hudson WW, Ricketts WA (1980) A strategy for the measurement of homophobia. J Homosex 5(4):357–372
10. Morin SF, Garfinkle EM (1978) Male homophobia. J Soc Issues 34(1):29–47
11. Weinstein N, Ryan WS, Dehaan CR, Przybylski AK, Legate N, Ryan RM (2012) Parental autonomy support and discrepancies between implicit and explicit sexual identities: dynamics of self-acceptance and defense. J Pers Soc Psychol 102:815–832
12. Thompson C, Zoloth B (1989) Homophobia. Campaign to End Homophobia, Cambridge, MA
13. Blumenfeld WJ (2000) How homophobia hurts everyone. In: Adams M, Blumenfeld WJ, Castañeda R, Hackman HW, Peters ML, Xúñiga X (eds) Readings for diversity and social justice: an anthology on racism, sexism, anti-semitism, heterosexism, classism and ableism. Routledge, New York, pp 267–275
14. Cowan G, Heiple B, Marquez C, Khatchadourian D, McNevin M (2005) Heterosexuals' attitudes toward hate crimes and hate speech against gays and lesbians: old-fashioned and modern heterosexism. J Homosex 49(2):67–82
15. Morrison MA, Morrison TG (2002) Development and validation of a scale measuring modern prejudice toward gay men and lesbian women. J Homosex 43(2):15–37
16. Raja S, Stokes JP (1998) Assessing attitudes toward lesbians and gay men: the modern homophobia scale. Int J Sex Gender Stud 3:113–134
17. Herek GM, Gillis JR, Cogan JC (2009) Internalized stigma among sexual minority adults: insights from a social psychological perspective. J Couns Psychol 56:32–43
18. Greenwald AG, McGhee DE, Schwartz JL (1998) Measuring individual differences in implicit cognition: the implicit association test. J Pers Soc Psychol 74:1464–1480
19. Banse R, Seise J, Zerbes N (2001) Implicit attitudes towards homosexuality: reliability, validity, and controllability of the IAT. Z Exp Psychol 48:145–160

20. Karpinski A, Steinman RB (2006) The single category implicit association test as a measure of implicit social cognition. J Pers Soc Psychol 91:16–32
21. Steffens MC, Buchner A (2003) Implicit Association Test: separating transsituationally stable and variable components of attitudes toward gay men. Exp Psychol 50:33–48
22. Costa AB, Bandeira DR, Nardi HC (2013) Systematic review of instruments measuring homophobia and related constructs. J Appl Soc Psychol 43:1324–1332
23. Lottes IL, Grollman EA (2010) Conceptualization and assessment of homonegativity. Int J Sex Health 22:219–233
24. Lingiardi V, Falanga S, D'Augelli AR (2005) The evaluation of homophobia in an Italian sample. Arch Sex Behav 34:81–93
25. Lingiardi V, Baiocco R, Nardelli N (2012) Measure of internalized sexual stigma for lesbians and gay men: a new scale. J Homosex 59:1191–1210
26. Rozin P, Haidt J, McCauley CR (2008) Disgust. In: Lewis M, Haviland-Jones JM, Barrett LF (eds) Handbook of emotions, 3rd edn. Guilford, New York, NY, pp 757–776
27. Navarrete CD, Fessler DM (2006) Disease avoidance and ethnocentrism: the effects of disease vulnerability and disgust sensitivity on intergroup attitudes. Evol Hum Behav 27:270–282
28. Hodson G, Costello K (2007) Interpersonal disgust, ideological orientations, and dehumanization as predictors of intergroup attitudes. Psychol Sci 18:691–698
29. Nussbaum MC (2010) From disgust to humanity: sexual orientation and constitutional law. Oxford University Press, New York, NY
30. Inbar Y, Pizarro DA, Bloom P (2012) Disgusting smells cause decreased liking of gay men. Emotion 12:23–27
31. Inbar Y, Pizarro DA, Knobe J, Bloom P (2009) Disgust sensitivity predicts intuitive disapproval of gays. Emotion 9:435–439
32. Schaller M, Park JH (2011) The behavioral immune system (and why it matters). Curr Dir Psychol Sci 20:99–103
33. Cullen JM, Wright LW Jr, Alessandri M (2002) The personality variable openness to experience as it relates to homophobia. J Homosex 42(4):119–134
34. Herek GM, Capitanio JP (1999) Sex differences in how heterosexuals think about lesbians and gay men: evidence from survey context effects. J Sex Res 36:348–360
35. Smith SJ, Axelton AM, Saucier DA (2009) The effects of contact on sexual prejudice: a meta-analysis. Sex Roles 61:178–191
36. Allport GW (1954) The nature of prejudice. Perseus Books, Cambridge, MA
37. Olson LR, Cadge W, Harrison JT (2006) Religion and public opinion about same-sex marriage. Soc Sci Q 87(2):340–360
38. Schwartz J (2010) Investigating differences in public support for gay rights issues. J Homosex 57:748–759
39. Herek GM (2002) Gender gaps in public opinion about lesbians and gay men. Public Opin Q 66:40–66
40. Kerns JG, Fine MA (1994) The relation between gender and negative attitudes toward gay men and lesbians: do gender role attitudes mediate this relation? Sex Roles 31:297–307
41. Kite ME (1984) Sex differences in attitudes toward homosexuals: a meta-analytic review. J Homosex 10(1–2):69–81
42. Kite ME, Whitley BE (1996) Sex differences in attitudes toward homosexual persons, behaviors, and civil rights: a meta-analysis. Pers Soc Psychol Bull 22:336–353
43. Parrott DJ, Adams HE, Zeichner A (2002) Homophobia: personality and attitudinal correlates. Pers Indiv Differ 32:1269–1278
44. Steffens MC, Wagner C (2004) Attitudes toward lesbians, gay men, bisexual women, and bisexual men in Germany. J Sex Res 41(2):137–149
45. Barron JM, Struckman-Johnson C, Quevillon R, Banka SR (2008) Heterosexual men's attitudes toward gay men: a hierarchical model including masculinity, openness, and theoretical explanations. Psychol Men Masculin 9:154–166

46. Shackelford TK, Besser A (2007) Predicting attitudes toward homosexuality: insights from personality psychology. Indiv Differ Res 5(2):106–114
47. Mays VM, Cochran SD (2001) Mental health correlates of perceived discrimination among lesbian, gay, and bisexual adults in the United States. Am J Public Health 91:1869–1876
48. Newcomb ME, Mustanski B (2010) Internalized homophobia and internalizing mental health problems: a meta-analytic review. Clin Psychol Rev 30:1019–1029
49. Rivers I (2011) Homophobic bullying: research and theoretical perspectives. Oxford University Press, New York, NY
50. Roberts AL, Austin SB, Corliss HL, Vandermorris AK, Koenen KC (2010) Pervasive trauma exposure among US sexual orientation minority adults and risk of posttraumatic stress disorder. Am J Public Health 100:2433–2441
51. Hatzenbuehler ML, O'Cleirigh C, Grasso C, Mayer K, Safren S, Bradford J (2012) Effect of same-sex marriage laws on health care use and expenditures in sexual minority men: a quasi-natural experiment. Am J Public Health 102:285–291
52. Hatzenbuehler ML, McLaughlin KA, Keyes KM, Hasin DS (2010) The impact of institutional discrimination on psychiatric disorders in lesbian, gay, and bisexual populations: a prospective study. Am J Public Health 100:452–459
53. Hatzenbuehler ML, Keyes KM, Hasin DS (2009) State-level policies and psychiatric morbidity in lesbian, gay, and bisexual populations. Am J Public Health 99:2275–2281
54. Hatzenbuehler ML, Pachankis JE, Wolff J (2012) Religious climate and health risk behaviors in sexual minority youths: a population-based study. Am J Public Health 102:657–663
55. Dragowski E, Halkitis P, Grossman A, D'Augelli A (2011) Sexual orientation victimization and posttraumatic stress symptoms among lesbian, gay, and bisexual youth. J Gay Lesbian Soc Serv 23:226–249
56. Meyer IH, Northridge ME (2007) The health of sexual minorities: public health perspectives on lesbian, gay, bisexual, transgender populations. Springer, New York, NY
57. Nadal KL, Issa MA, Leon J, Meterko V, Wideman M, Wong Y (2011) Sexual orientation microaggressions: "death by a thousand cuts" for lesbian, gay, and bisexual youth. J LGBT Youth 8:234–259
58. Hatzenbuehler ML (2009) How does sexual minority stigma "get under the skin"? A psychological mediation framework. Psychol Bull 135:707–730
59. Meyer IH (1995) Minority stress and mental health in gay men. J Health Soc Behav 36(1):38–56
60. Meyer IH (2003) Prejudice, social stress, and mental health in lesbian, gay, and bisexual populations: conceptual issues and research evidence. Psychol Bull 129:674–697
61. Frost DM, Meyer IH (2009) Internalized homophobia and relationship quality among lesbians, gay men, and bisexuals. J Couns Psychol 56:97–109
62. Lingiardi V, Nardelli N (2012) Partner relational problem: listening beyond homo-ignorance and homo-prejudice. In: Levounis P, Drescher J, Barber ME (eds) The LGBT casebook. American Psychiatric Publishing, Washington, DC, pp 223–230
63. Balsam DM, Szymanski KF (2005) Insidious trauma: examining the relationship between heterosexism and lesbians' PTSD symptoms. Traumatology 17(2):4–13
64. Bartholomew K, Regan KV, Oram D, White MA (2008) Correlates of partner abuse in male same-sex relationships. Violence Vict 23:344–360
65. Carvalho A, Lewis R, Derlega V, Winstead B, Viggiano C (2011) Internalized sexual minority stressors and same-sex intimate partner violence. J Fam Violence 26:501–509
66. Drescher J (1998) Psychoanalytic therapy and the gay man. The Analytic, London
67. Isay RA (1989) Being homosexual: gay men and their development. Farrar, Straus, Giroux, New York, NY
68. Drescher J (2012) What's in your closet? In: Levounis P, Drescher J, Barber ME (eds) The LGBT casebook. American Psychiatric Publishing, Washington, DC, pp 3–16

69. Cohen KM, Savin-Williams RC (2012) Coming out to self and others: developmental milestones. In: Levounis P, Drescher J, Barber ME (eds) The LGBT casebook. American Psychiatric Publishing, Washington, DC, pp 17–33
70. Murray CE, Mobley AK (2009) Empirical research about same-sex intimate partner violence: a methodological review. J Homosex 56:361–386
71. Balsam KF (2001) Nowhere to hide: lesbian battering, homophobia, and minority stress. Women Ther 23(3):25–37
72. Browning C (1995) Silence on same-sex partner abuse. Alternate Routes 12:95–106
73. Murray CE, Mobley AK, Buford AP, Seaman-DeJohn MM (2006/2007) Same-sex intimate partner violence: dynamics, social context, and counseling implications. J LGBT Issues Couns 1(4):7–30
74. Telesco GA (2003) Sex role identity and jealousy as correlates of abusive behavior in lesbian relationships. J Hum Behav Soc Environ 8:153–169
75. Sue DW (2010) Microaggressions in everyday life: race, gender, and sexual orientation. Wiley, Hoboken
76. D'Augelli AR, Pilkington NW, Hershberger SL (2002) Incidence and mental health impact of sexual orientation victimization of lesbian, gay, and bisexual youths in high school. Sch Psychol Q 17:148–167
77. Rivers I (2004) Recollections of bullying at school and their long-term implications for lesbians, gay men, and bisexuals. Crisis 25:169–175
78. Robinson JP, Espelage DL (2012) Inequities in educational and psychological outcomes between LGBTQ and straight students in middle and high school. Educ Res 40:315–330
79. Birkett M, Espelage DL, Koenig B (2009) LGB and questioning students in schools: the moderating effects of homophobic bullying and school climate on negative outcomes. J Youth Adolesc 38:989–1000
80. Holt MK, Matjasko JL, Espelage D, Reid G, Koenig B (2013) Sexual risk taking and bullying among adolescents. Pediatrics 132:e1481–e1487
81. Espelage DL, Basile KC, Hamburger ME (2012) Bullying perpetration and subsequent sexual violence perpetration among middle school students. J Adolesc Health 50:60–65
82. Marshal MP, Dietz LJ, Friedman MS, Stall R, Smith HA, McGinley J, Thoma BC, Murray PJ, D'Augelli AR, Brent DA (2011) Suicidality and depression disparities between sexual minority and heterosexual youth: a meta-analytic review. J Adolesc Health 49:115–123
83. Ryan C, Huebner D, Diaz RM, Sanchez J (2009) Family rejection as a predictor of negative health outcomes in white and Latino lesbian, gay, and bisexual young adults. Pediatrics 123:346–352
84. Baiocco R, Laghi F, Di Pomponio I, Nigito CS (2012) Self-disclosure to the best friend: friendship quality and internalized sexual stigma in Italian lesbian and gay adolescents. J Adolesc 35:381–387
85. UN News Service (2011) Homophobic bullying represents grave violation of human rights – Ban (8 December 2011). http://www.un.org/apps/news/story.asp?NewsID=40671. Accessed 15 Jan 2014
86. UNESCO (2011) Rio Statement on homophobic bullying and education for all (10 December 2011). http://www.unesco.org/new/en/hiv-and-aids/our-priorities-in-hiv/gender-equality/anti-bullying/. Accessed 15 Jan 2014
87. Poteat VP, Russell ST (2013) Understanding homophobic behavior and its implications for policy and practice. Theory Pract 52:264–271
88. Finneran C, Stephenson R (2013) Gay and bisexual men's perceptions of police helpfulness in response to male-male intimate partner violence. J Homosex 14:354–362. doi:10.5811/westjem.2013.3.15639
89. Berrill KT, Herek GM (1990) Primary and secondary victimization in anti-gay hate crimes official response and public policy. J Interpers Violence 5:401–413
90. Brown SL (2007) Counseling victims of violence: a handbook for helping professionals, 2nd edn. Hunter House, Alameda, CA

91. Drescher J (2010) Queer diagnoses: parallels and contrasts in the history of homosexuality, gender variance, and the diagnostic and statistical manual. Arch Sex Behav 39:427–460
92. Bartlett A, Smith G, King M (2009) The response of mental health professionals to clients seeking help to change or redirect same-sex sexual orientation. BMC Psychiatry 9:11. doi:10.1186/1471-244X-9-11
93. Lingiardi V, Capozzi P (2004) Psychoanalytic attitudes towards homosexuality: an empirical research. Int J Psychoanal 85:137–157
94. APA Task Forceon Appropriate Therapeutic Responses to Sexual Orientation (2009) Report of the task force on appropriate therapeutic responses to sexual orientation. American Psychological Association, Washington, DC
95. Pan American Health Organization, Regional Office of the WHO (2012) "Cures" for an illness that does not exist: purported therapies aimed at changing sexual orientation lack medical justification and are ethically unacceptable. http://www.paho.org/hq/index.php?option=com_docman&task=doc_view&gid=17703. Accessed 15 Jan 2014
96. Lingiardi V, Nardelli N (2014) Linee guida per la consulenza psicologica e la psicoterapia con persone lesbiche, gay, bisessuali [Guidelines for psychological counseling and psychotherapy with lesbians, gay men, and bisexuals]. Raffaello Cortina, Milan
97. Shidlo A, Schroeder M (2002) Changing sexual orientation: a consumers' report. Prof Psychol Res Pract 33:249
98. Spitzer RL (2012) Spitzer reassesses his 2003 study of reparative therapy of homosexuality. Arch Sex Behav 41:757
99. Baiocco R, Argalia M, Laghi F (2012) The desire to marry and attitudes toward same-sex family legalization in a sample of Italian lesbians and gay men. J Fam Issues 35:181–200
100. Baiocco R, Ioverno S, Lonigro A, Baumgartner E, Laghi F (2014) Suicidal ideation among Italian and Spanish young adults: the role of sexual orientation. Arch Suicide Res. doi:10.1080/13811118.2013.833150

Transphobia

Elisa Bandini and Mario Maggi

4.1 Background and Definitions

According to DSM-V [1], "*transgender* refers to the broad spectrum of individuals who transiently or persistently identify with a gender different from their natal gender."

The term *transphobia* has been defined as "emotional disgust toward individuals who do not conform to society's gender expectations," such as masculine women, feminine men, cross-dressers, or transgenders [2]; this definition is specular with Weinberg's classic definition of homophobia [3].

In addition to transphobia (the attitudinal component), Hill suggested two more components to conceptualize hate against transgenders: genderism, which reflects the cognitive component, and genderbashing, referring to the behavioral component. In particular, *genderism* is a social system of beliefs that reinforces the negative evaluation of individuals not conforming to the society's gender role expectations. *Genderbashing* refers to behaviors of harassment and/or physical assault of individuals not conforming to society's gender norms [4]. More recently, Sugano et al. have proposed that the term transphobia "refers to societal discrimination and stigma of individuals who do not conform to traditional norms of sex and gender" (p. 217) [5].

The classic starting point for defining the *stigma* is the presence of a characteristic which the individual possesses or is believed to possess "that is deeply discrediting" [6]. The recognition of this characteristic leads the stigmatized person to be deeply devalued in a particular social context [7].

Three components of stigma have been described:
1. Perceived stigma, referred to the belief of a potential stigmatized individual when society holds a negative attitude toward his/her group of persons [8].

E. Bandini • M. Maggi (✉)
Sexual Medicine and Andrology Unit, Department of Experimental, Clinical and Biomedical Sciences, University of Florence, Viale Pieraccini 6, Florence 50139, Italy
e-mail: elisa.bandini.psy@gmail.com; m.maggi@dfc.unifi.it

It includes also how the individual thinks society views him/her personally as a member of the stigmatized group [9].
2. Experienced stigma, referred to as the "experience of actual discrimination and/or participation restrictions on the part of the person affected" [8].
3. Self-stigma, characterized by feelings of shame, loss of self-esteem, hopelessness, guilt deriving from the adoption of a stigmatized view of oneself [10].

Stigma has been also defined as an overarching term which includes ignorance/misinformation (problem of knowledge), prejudice (problem of attitude), and discrimination (problem of behavior) [11].

4.2 The Expressions of Transphobia

While a large amount of literature on homophobia has been produced, transphobia remains an understudied topic.

Moreover, the majority of the studies available do not distinguish transgenders from the gay, lesbian, and bisexual (LGB) population and do not address the differences between gender role, gender identity, and sexual orientation. In fact, transgenders are outside the male/female gender binary, whereas LGB individuals are outside the expected heterosexual identity [12]. However, both populations are challenging the male–female dichotomy and share some prejudice mechanisms [13].

Recently, a growing body of research has documented the presence of *prejudice, discrimination, harassment, violence, and hate crimes* against transgenders, as reported below [4, 14–19].

4.2.1 Prejudice

The term ***prejudice*** refers to preconceived, usually unfavorable, judgments toward people or a person because of personal characteristics (such as gender, social class, age, disability, religion, sexuality, race/ethnicity, language, nationality) [20].

Understanding the mechanisms of prejudices is important in order to reduce their harm through psychoeducational, clinical, and social interventions.

Despite research on this topic being just at the beginning, in recent years some measures to assess anti-transgender prejudice have been developed [2, 21–23] and used to compare the extent of this attitude in different samples [24, 25].

Gender differences have been assessed, with women reporting a less negative attitude than men [2, 18, 21, 26, 27]. Also gay men display higher transphobia than lesbians [12]. It has been speculated that the higher level of prejudice experienced by men is linked to the greater threat to their dominant social role [21].

Moreover, prejudice against transgenders is correlated with anti-lesbian and gay prejudice [2, 13, 21]. This finding is consistent with society's perception of LGBTQ (gay, lesbian, bisexual, transgender, queer) as a group that violates traditional gender role prescriptions [28]. Coherently, also traditional gender role attitudes and beliefs constitute an important correlate of both anti-transgender [2, 13, 29, 30] and anti-LGB prejudice [31, 32]. Therefore, both anti-LGB prejudice and traditional gender role attitudes seem to be important targets in interventions aiming to mitigate transphobia [13].

Furthermore, in a recent empirical research aimed at elucidating the constellation of constructs associated with prejudice against transgenders, Tebbe et al. found a unique association of anti-transgenders prejudice with a "need for closure" [13]. The latter is defined as a person's desire for structure, order, and non-ambiguity [33]; therefore a high need for closure will bring the person to avoid uncertainty, or anything threatening the ability to attain cognitive closure [34]. In fact, individuals with a high need for closure display a negative attitude toward groups who disrupt existing social categories, such as LGB [35, 36] and transgenders [13]. Moreover, in a multisite and multi-study investigation, assessing samples from Canada, the United States, and the Philippines, intolerance toward transgenders was associated also with social conformism, religious fundamentalism, moral dogmatism, ego-defensiveness, authoritarian beliefs, and low self-esteem [37].

When differences in the transgender group are accounted for, transsexuals seem to evoke a reasonably good attitude in comparison with other groups which do not display a binary gender role [22, 26]. This finding is not surprising, because transsexuals tend to reproduce the binary model of gender, rather than subvert it. In fact, according to DSM-V [1], the term *transsexual* denotes an individual who seeks, or has undergone, a social transition from male to female or female to male, which usually also involves a somatic transition by cross-sex hormone treatment and genital surgery.

4.2.2 Discrimination and Harassment

Discrimination is the prejudicial treatment of an individual based on his actual or perceived membership in a certain group or category, often leading him to isolation [38, 39].

The term ***harassment*** covers a wide range of behaviors of an offensive nature, aimed to disturb or upset.

Transgenders face persistent and intense discrimination across various life domains. A troubling array of difficulties were reported, such as economical discrimination, experiences of harassment at home, work, school, and discrimination by government agencies, medical professionals, and other service providers [37, 40, 41].

The European Union Agency for Fundamental Rights (FRA) [42] has recently conducted online the EU (European Union) LGBT survey in the 27 EU Member States and Croatia, collecting the responses from more than 93,000 LGBT persons. This survey is the largest of its kind to date and represents the most wide ranging and comprehensive picture available of the experience of LGBT people residing in these countries. Transgender respondents reported that they experience an environment less tolerant toward them than that which was reported by LGB respondents. They are, for instance, the most likely of all LGBT subgroups to report personal discrimination in the past year because of being LGBT, particularly in the areas of employment and health care. In particular, 29 % of the transgender respondents who were employed and/or looking for a job in the 12 months before the survey felt discriminated against in these situations in the past year. This was more than twice the equivalent percentage of LGB respondents [42].

In addition to the aforementioned observations, a national Dutch survey reported that 42 % received negative reactions because of their transgender identity, most commonly in public (38 %) and at work or school (21 %) [43].

Regarding US data, a survey of 6,450 transgender and gender nonconforming respondents from all 50 American states revealed that 47 % reported an adverse job outcome, 29 % police disrespect or harassment, and 15 % of students dropped out of school as a result of severe harassment [44]. More recently, in a national study of the US transgender population, 70 % of individuals reported experience of verbal abuse and harassment related to being transgender and 38 % employment discrimination [45].

4.2.3 Violence

Violence, physical and verbal victimization, and sexual assault motivated by the gender identity of the victim are widespread, although the exact extent cannot be known [14, 15, 46].

According to the FRA (2013 EU LGBT survey) [42], LGBT respondents are subject to high levels of repeated victimization and violence, which is especially high for transgenders. In particular, in the last 5 years, 35 % of all transgender respondents had been attacked or threatened with violence at home or elsewhere. Moreover, 22 % of all transgenders reported to have been, in the year before the survey, victims of harassment, perceived partly or completely happened because they are LGBT. Finally, about 3 in 10 (28 %) of all transgenders said they were victims of violence or threats of violence more than three times in the past year [42].

4.2.4 Hate Crimes

It is well established that sexual minorities experience hate crimes [47]. A *hate crime* is defined as an "unlawful, violent, destructive or threatening conduct in which the perpetrator is motivated by prejudice toward the victim's putative social group." [48]. According to the Federal Bureau of Investigation, 17.4 % of the hate crimes perpetuated between 1995 and 2008 targeted sexual minorities [49]; this rate, as highlighted by Duncan [50], is more than eight times what would be expected considering the relatively low percentage of sexual minorities in the general population.

The most shocking expression of transphobia is the murder of hundreds of transgenders across the world, as documented by the latest records of deaths provided by the Transgender Europe network (TGEU) on 12 March, 2013, in the framework of its Trans Murder Monitoring Project [51]. According to such records, 1,123 transgenders were murdered in 57 countries worldwide from January 1st, 2008 to December 31st, 2012. The reports show a constant increase in reported killings of transgenders over the last 5 years, most of them in Central and South America. Moreover, it has to be considered that this number may be underestimated because in most countries data on these murders are not recorded systematically [51]. According to the TGEU, 20 transgenders have been murdered between 2008 and March 2013 in Italy [51].

4.3 The Impact of Transphobia

A large body of evidence demonstrates the effect of stigma in affecting feelings, attitudes, and behavior of both the person affected and family members [52]. In particular, lower self-esteem, poorer self-care, and social isolation have been linked with experienced stigma [9].

Moreover, stigma has a corrosive influence on health, through its influence on self-esteem, coping behaviors, social relationships, and material resources [53].

The negative impact of transphobia on the lives of transgenders has also been documented [14, 15, 27]. As recently reported by Amnesty International [46], because of prejudice, discrimination, and violence, many transgenders in Europe continue to hide their gender identity. For instance, according to a survey published by FRA, almost 70 % of the European LGBT respondents had always or often disguised their sexual orientation or gender identity at school [42]. Furthermore, from a study based on transgenders interviews [16], it emerges that the most common theme for the individuals interviewed was a stated desire for acceptance, to simply be known as just another person.

What is more, transphobia may be involved in the high rates of psychological distress and suicidal tendencies observed among transgenders [14, 54].

4.3.1 The Impact of Transphobia on General Health

According to FRA [42], European transgenders who had accessed healthcare or social services in the last 12 months display a level of discrimination twice as high as the LGB population; in particular, around one in five said they felt discriminated against by healthcare (19 %) or social services (17 %) personnel in the year before the survey.

The health inequities experienced by this population have negative health impacts that include increased risks for chronic disease and mental health concerns [53]. In fact, past and/or repeated experiences of discrimination by the healthcare system may constitute a powerful deterrent to seeking treatment [5, 19, 41].

Another factor linking stigma with poor health status is social isolation [55]. High levels of social isolation have been observed in various stigmatized groups, including sexual minorities [55].

Moreover, stigma is associated with more maladaptive coping behavior and higher level of stress, which in turn are linked with adverse health outcomes [53].

4.3.2 The Impact of Transphobia on Mental Health

Stigma has a tremendous negative impact on the victims' lives. For instance, they may feel unsure regarding how "normal" persons will judge them [6] and always wondering what impression they are making [56]. Moreover, stigma is associated with maladaptive emotion regulation strategies which in turn produce greater psychological distress [53] and with maladaptive coping behaviors (such as smoking and drinking) [57] that increase the risk for adverse health outcomes.

Minority stress model [58] has been proposed and tested to explain the association between stigma and mental health. This theory postulates that stigma attached to one's minority status adds stress beyond general stress that individuals normally face. This added stress in turn negatively affects general and mental health. Both external events, such as victimization and violence, and internal responses, such as expectations of rejection, constitute minority stress, and both are associated with health problems [58].

Transgenders display low self-esteem and social isolation, together with high rates of lifetime depression, and suicidal ideation and attempts [59, 60]. Just recently several studies have been concentrated on testing the presence of an association between transphobia and mental health. In particular, it has been demonstrated that transphobia is significantly associated with current depression [14, 61] and suicidal risk [62]. In a recent study, Duncan et al. [50] reported that sexual-minority youths residing in neighborhoods with higher rates of LGBT assault hate crimes were significantly more likely to report suicidal ideation and attempts than were those residing in neighborhoods with lower LGBT assault hate crime rates.

Nuttbrock et al. [63] found, in a sample of transgender women, a strong association between gender-related abuse and depression. This seems to be particularly true in the early stages of life, possibly due to the development of coping mechanisms later in life [63]. In fact, resiliency factors may improve the detrimental effect of stigma on mental health. Interestingly, Bockting et al. [45] have tested three factors of resilience (identity pride, family support, and transgender peer support) in a large Internet-based sample of the US transgender population. Using a standardized instrument, they observed that 49 % of transgender women and 37 % of transgender men reported clinical levels of depression and 33 % of each gender group reported anxiety. Both experienced and perceived stigma were positively associated with overall psychological distress. Moreover, identity pride and family support were both negatively associated with psychological distress, but only transgender peer support was a protective factor for mental health [45]. In fact, a community of peers not only provides a space where one is not stigmatized, but also offers an alternative reference group to evaluate oneself in comparison to similar others.

4.3.3 The Impact of Transphobia on Transgender Identity Development

The impact of stigma in shaping mental health, resilience, and identity depends greatly on the age when it is experienced. Regarding transgenders, it is well established that experiencing stigma at an early age increases the risk of isolation, academic performance problems and school dropout, homelessness, substance abuse, and suicide in gender nonconforming youth [64, 65]. On the other hand, this youth can also have the opportunity to develop early resilience, and, as pointed out by Bockting [66], can easily develop a coherent sense of self, because their gender identity is noticed and mirrored by the society. In contrast, youth who are not yet expressing a nonconforming gender can experience more difficulties in the development of their transgender identity; in fact, they may live hiding their gender identity according to the external expectations. Therefore, they do not have any external confirmation of their identity and thus may result in mental health (for instance, obsessive/compulsive symptoms related to cross-dressing and gender dysphoria) and identity difficulties [66].

4.4 European Legislation

Despite standards on nondiscrimination and equality for LGBT persons having been further developed by the European Union (EU), the Council of Europe, and the United Nations (UN), high rates of discrimination, harassment, and violence are still experienced by this population [67–69]. Moreover, the EU FRA survey shows very high non-reporting rates among respondents who had experienced transphobia. The most frequent reasons for not reporting incidents of discrimination were a belief that "nothing would change," and a lack of knowledge about how or where to report it [42]. Therefore, it is important to develop strategies aimed at improving rights awareness and reporting discrimination and violence.

Physical violence targeting individuals on the grounds of their gender identity are hate crimes. The discriminatory nature of the motive sets hate crimes apart from other criminal acts. These attacks violate several human rights, such as the right to human dignity (Article 1 of the EU Charter of Fundamental Rights), the right to life (Article 2 of the EU Charter), and the right to the integrity of the person and protection from violence (Article 3 of the EU Charter) [70]. Unfortunately, according to the Organization for Security and Cooperation in Europe (OSCE) only five EU countries collect data on transphobic hate crimes [71]. Moreover, several States did not yet explicate in their legislation that a crime perpetrated on the grounds of real or perceived sexual orientation or gender identity constitutes a hate crime. Also the EU lacks an adequate legislation.

According to Amnesty International [46], States should comprehensively address hate crimes by adopting legislation to prohibit them. Furthermore, crimes perpetrated on the basis of sexual orientation or gender identity should be considered hate crimes. States should also ensure that the law is applied in practice and should collect thorough data on these forms of crimes in order to adopt and implement robust policies aimed at eliminating discrimination and promoting equality.

References

1. American Psychiatric Association (2013) Diagnostic and statistical manual of mental disorders, 5th edn: DSM-5 tm. American Psychiatric Association, Washington, DC
2. Hill DB, Willoughby BLB (2005) The development and validation of the genderism and transphobia scale. Sex Roles 53:531–544
3. Weinberg G (1972) Society and the healthy homosexual. St. Martins Press, New York, NY
4. Hill DB (2002) Genderism, transphobia, and gender bashing: a framework for interpreting anti-transgender violence. In: Wallace B, Carter R (eds) Understanding and dealing with violence: a multicultural approach. Sage, Thousand Oaks, CA, pp 113–136
5. Sugano E, Nemoto T, Operario D (2006) The impact of exposure to transphobia on HIV risk behavior in a sample of transgendered women of color in San Franscisco. AIDS Behav 10:217–225
6. Goffman E (1963) Stigma: notes on the management of spoiled identity. Penguin, London
7. Crocker J, Major B, Steele C (1998) Social stigma. In: Gilbert DT, Fiske ST, Lindzey G (eds) Handbook of social psychology. McGraw-Hill, Boston, MA, pp 504–533
8. Van Brakel WH, Anderson AM, Mutatkar RK et al (2006) The participation scale: measuring a key concept in public health. Disabil Rehabil 28:193–203
9. LeBel T (2008) Perceptions of and responses to stigma. Soc Compass 2:409–432
10. Yanos PT, Roe D, Markus K et al (2008) Pathways between internalised stigma and outcomes related to recovery in schizophrenia spectrum disorders. Psychiatr Serv 59:1437–1442
11. Thornicroft G, Rose D, Kassam A et al (2007) Stigma: ignorance, prejudice or discrimination? Br J Psychiatry 190:192–193
12. Warriner K, Nagoshi CT, Nagoshi JL (2013) Correlates of homophobia, transphobia, and internalized homophobia in gay or lesbian and heterosexual samples. J Homosex 60:1297–1314
13. Tebbe EN, Moradi B (2012) Anti-transgender prejudice: a structural equation model of associated constructs. J Couns Psychol 59:251–261
14. Clements-Nolle K, Marx R, Katz M (2006) Attempted suicide among transgender persons: the influence of gender-based discrimination and victimization. J Homosex 51:53–69
15. Lombardi EL, Wilchins R, Priesing D et al (2001) Gender violence: transgender experiences with violence and discrimination. J Homosex 42:89–101
16. Gagne P, Tewksbury R, McGaughey D (1996) Coming out and crossing over: identity formation and proclamation in the transgender community. Gend Soc 11:478–508
17. Grossman AH, D'Augelli AR (2006) Transgender youth: invisible and vulnerable. J Homosex 51:111–128
18. Tee N, Hegarty P (2006) Predicting opposition to the civil rights of transpersons in the United Kingdom. J Community Appl Soc Psychol 16:70–80
19. Xavier JM, Simmons R (2000) The Washington transgender needs assessment survey. http://www.glaa.org/archive/2000/tgneedsassessment1112.shtml. Accessed Mar 2014

20. Dovidio JF, Gaertner SL (2010) Intergroup bias. In: Fiske ST, Gilbert DT, Lindzey G (eds) The handbook of social psychology, vol 2, 5th edn. Wiley, New York, NY
21. Nagoshi JL, Adams KA, Terrell HK et al (2008) Gender differences in correlates of homophobia and transphobia. Sex Roles 59:521–531
22. Carrera-Fernández MV, Lameiras-Fernández M, Rodríguez-Castro Y, et al (2013) Spanish adolescents' attitudes toward transpeople: proposal and validation of a short form of the genderism and transphobia scale. J Sex Res [Epub ahead of print]
23. Walch SE, Ngamake ST, Francisco J et al (2012) The attitudes toward transgendered individuals scale: psychometric properties. Arch Sex Behav 41:1283–1291
24. Gerhardstein KR, Anderson VN (2010) There's more than meets the eye: facial appearance and evaluations of transsexual people. Sex Roles 62:361–373
25. Hill DB, Menvielle E, Sica KM et al (2010) An affirmative intervention for families with gender variant children: parental ratings of child mental health and gender. J Sex Marital Ther 36:6–23
26. Landen M, Innala S (2000) Attitudes toward transsexualism in a Swedish national survey. Arch Sex Behav 29:375–388
27. Winter S, Webster B, Cheung PKE (2008) Measuring Hong Kong undergraduate students' attitudes towards transpeople. Sex Roles 59:670–683
28. Fassinger RE, Arseneau JR (2007) "I'd rather get wet than be under that umbrella": differentiating the experiences and identities of lesbian, gay, bisexual, and transgender people. In: Bieschke KJ, Perez RM, DeBord KA (eds) Handbook of counseling and psychotherapy with lesbian, gay, bisexual, and transgender clients. American Psychological Association, Washington, DC, pp 19–49
29. Lombardi EL (2009) Varieties of transgender/transsexual lives and their relationship with transphobia. J Homosex 56:977–992
30. Nadal K, Rivera D, Corpus M (2010) Sexual orientation and transgender microaggressions: implications for mental health and counseling. In: Sue DW (ed) Microaggressions and marginality: manifestation, dynamics, and impact. Wiley, Hoboken, NJ, pp 217–240
31. Goodman MB, Moradi B (2008) Attitudes and behaviors toward lesbians and gay men: critical correlates and mediated relations. J Couns Psychol 55:371–384
32. Herek GM (2002) Heterosexuals' attitudes toward bisexual men and women in the United States. J Sex Res 39:264–274
33. Webster DM, Kruglanski AW (1994) Individual differences in need for cognitive closure. J Pers Soc Psychol 67:1049–1062
34. Kruglanski AW (1990) Motivations for judging and knowing: implications for causal attribution. In: Higgins ET, Sorrentino RM (eds) The handbook of motivation and cognition: foundation of social behavior. Guilford, New York, NY, pp 333–368
35. Haslam N, Rothschild L, Ernst D (2002) Are essentialist beliefs associated with prejudice? Br J Soc Psychol 41:87–100
36. Mohr JJ, Rochlen AB (1999) Measuring attitudes regarding bisexuality in lesbian, gay male, and heterosexual populations. J Couns Psychol 46:353–369
37. Willoughby BLB, Hill DB, Gonzalez CA et al (2010) Who hates gender outlaws? A multisite and multinational evaluation of the genderism and transphobia scale. Int J Transgend 12(4):254–271
38. "Discrimination, definition". Cambridge Dictionaries Online. Cambridge University, p 346. http://dictionary.cambridge.org/dictionary/british/discrimination_1. Accessed Mar 2014
39. Appelbaum RP, Duneier M, Giddens A (2009) Introduction to sociology, 7th edn. W. W. Norton, New York, p 334
40. Whittle S, Turner L, Al-Alami M (2007) Engendered penalties: transgendered and transsexual people's experiences of inequality and discrimination. Manchester Metropolitan University and Press for Change, Manchester
41. Kosenko K, Rintamaki L, Raney S et al (2013) Transgender patient perceptions of stigma in health care contexts. Med Care 51:819–822

42. FRA (2013) EU LGBT survey – European Union lesbian, gay, bisexual and transgender survey – main results, Luxembourg, Publications Office. Available at: http://fra.europa.eu/en/publication/2013/eu-lgbt-survey-main-results
43. Keuzenkamp S (2012) Worden wie je bent: Het leven van transgenders in Nederland. Sociaal en Cultureel Planbureau, Den Haag
44. Grant JM, Mottet LA, Tanis J et al (2011) Injustice at every turn: a report of the national transgender discrimination survey. National Center for Transgender Equality and National Gay and Lesbian Task Force, Washington, DC
45. Bockting WO, Miner MH, Swinburne RE et al (2013) Stigma, mental health, and resilience among an online sample of the U.S. transgender population. Am J Public Health 103:943–951
46. Amnesty International (2013) Because of who I am. Homophobia, transphobia and hate crimes in Europe. September 2013. Retrieved from http://www.amnesty.eu/content/assets/PressReleases/European_hate_crime_briefing.pdf
47. Herek GM (2009) Hate crimes and stigma-related experiences among sexual minority adults in the United States: prevalence estimates from a national probability sample. J Interpers Violence 24:54–74
48. Green DP, McFalls LH, Smith JK (2001) Hate crime: an emergent research agenda. Annu Rev Sociol 27:479–504
49. Federal Bureau of Investigation. Hate crimes. Available at: http://www.fbi.gov/about-us/cjis/ucr/hate-crime
50. Duncan DT, Hatzenbuehler ML (2014) Lesbian, gay, bisexual, and transgender hate crimes and suicidality among a population-based sample of sexual-minority adolescents in Boston. Am J Public Health 104:272–278
51. TvT research project (2013) Trans Murder Monitoring results: TMM MARCH 2013 Update, Transrespect versus Transphobia Worldwide (TvT) project website: http://www.transrespect-transphobia.org/en/tvt-project/tmm-results/march-2013.htm
52. Thornicroft G, Brohan E, Rose D et al (2009) Global pattern of experienced and anticipated discrimination against people with schizophrenia: a cross-sectional survey. Lancet 373:408–415
53. Hatzenbuehler ML, Phelan JC, Link BG (2013) Stigma as a fundamental cause of population health inequalities. Am J Public Health 103:813–821
54. Bockting W, Huang CY, Ding H et al (2005) Are transgender persons at higher risk for HIV than other sexual minorities? A comparison of HIV prevalence and risks. Int J Transgend 8:123–131
55. Hatzenbuehler ML, Nolen-Hoeksema S, Dovidio J (2009) How does stigma "get under the skin"? The mediating role of emotion regulation. Psychol Sci 20:1282–1289
56. Rush LL (1998) Affective reactions to multiple social stigmas. J Soc Psychol 138:421–430
57. Pachankis JE, Hatzenbuehler ML, Starks TJ (2014) The influence of structural stigma and rejection sensitivity on young sexual minority men's daily tobacco and alcohol use. Soc Sci Med 103:67–75
58. Meyer IH (2003) Prejudice, social stress, and mental health in lesbian, gay, and bisexual populations: conceptual issues and research evidence. Psychol Bull 129:674–697
59. Clements-Nolle K, Marx R, Guzman R et al (2001) HIV prevalence, risk behaviors, health care use, and mental health status of transgender persons: implications for public health intervention. Am J Public Health 91:915–921
60. Dean L, Meyer IH, Robinson K et al (2000) Lesbian, gay, bisexual, and transgender health: findings and concerns. J Gay Lesbian Med Assoc 4:102–151
61. Rotondi NK, Bauer GR, Travers R et al (2011) Depression in male-to-female transgender Ontarians: results from the Trans PULSE project. Can J Commun Ment Health 30:113–133
62. Marshal MP, Dietz LJ, Friedman MS et al (2011) Suicidality and depression disparities between sexual minority and heterosexual youth: a meta-analytic review. J Adolesc Health 49:115–123

63. Nuttbrock L, Hwahng S, Bockting W et al (2010) Psychiatric impact of gender-related abuse across the life course of male-to-female transgender persons. J Sex Res 47:12–23
64. Garofalo R, Deleon J, Osmer E, Doll M, Harper GW (2006) Overlooked, misunderstood and at-risk: exploring the lives and HIV risk of ethnic minority male-to-female transgender youth. J Adolesc Health 38:230–236
65. Grossman AH, D'Augelli AR (2007) Transgender youth and life-threatening behaviors. Suicide Life Threat Behav 37:527–537
66. Bockting W (2014) The impact of stigma on transgender identity development and mental health. In: Kreukels BPC, Steensma TD, de Vries ALC (eds) Gender dysphoria and disorders of sex development. Progress in care and knowledge. Springer, New York, NY, pp 319–330
67. REPORT on the EU Roadmap against homophobia and discrimination on grounds of sexual orientation and gender identity (2013/2183(INI)) Committee on Civil Liberties, Justice and Home Affairs. http://www.europarl.europa.eu/sides/getDoc.do?type=REPORT&reference=A7-2014-0009&language=EN
68. Council of Europe (2011) Discrimination on grounds of sexual orientation and gender identity in Europe, 2nd edn. Council of Europe Publishing, Paris. https://www.coe.int/t/commissioner/Source/LGBT/LGBTStudy2011_en.pdf. Accessed Mar 2014
69. United Nations (2011) The United Nations speaks out: tackling discrimination on grounds of sexual orientation and gender identity [Brochure]. Retrieved from http://www.ohchr.org/EN/Issues/Discrimination/Pages/LGBTBrochure.aspx
70. European Union (2010) Charter of Fundamental Rights of the European Union (2010/C 83/02). Official Journal of the European Union of 30 March 2010, pp 389–403. Retrieved from http://eur-lex.europa.eu/legal-content/EN/TXT/?uri=CELEX:12010P
71. ILGA Europe (2013) Violence against lesbian, gay, bisexual, transgender and intersex people in the OSCE region. Country-by-country information. Sources: submissions and reports by ILGA-Europe and its members. Retrieved from http://file:///C:/Users/Bartolini/Downloads/PUBLICVERSION-OSCE%20Hate%20Crime%20submission%202013mar31%20www.pdf

Sexual Abuse and Sexual Function

Alessandra H. Rellini

Awareness of child sexual abuse emerged along with the gaining of civil rights for children [1, 2]. In 1975, enough clinicians, mental health providers, and policy makers became aware of the alarmingly high rates of childhood abuse and neglect for an international conference on this topic to convene. Scholars were particularly concerned to learn that many mental health patients experienced sexual abuse, defined as forced and often traumatic sexual experiences, prior to age 16, a developmental time when the individual is still forming a sense of the sexual self [3]. The initial clinical observations of the relationship between childhood sexual abuse and negative psychiatric health have been confirmed by carefully executed epidemiological studies. At the present time, scholars agree that approximately 20 % of women in the USA have experienced a forced or coerced sexual experience prior to age 16 and 10 % of men have experienced a forced sexual experience at some point in their lives [4]. The definition of sexual experiences varies by study, but it usually involves the touching or penetration of genitals or rectum. The World Health Organization has adopted a much more broad definition of sexual violence and has included sexual harassment, but we will not include sexual harassment in our discussion of sexual abuse because the research on this topic is only in the beginning of its conception and, at this time, it is unclear about the similarity between the outcomes of abuse and harassment. Studies in other countries report more mixed results regarding the prevalence of sexual abuse; however, there is reason to believe that numbers are comparable. For example, in our work at a gynecology clinic in a small northern Italian town we found that 18 % of patients responded positively when asked about sexual abuse as part of confidential questionnaires (Rellini and Nappi, unpublished data). Similarly, in Sweden scholars estimated 12 % of women have experienced sexual abuse during childhood [5].

These numbers may seem unreasonable high at first glance, but they make sense once we take into consideration the larger social picture. A study of college men

A.H. Rellini (✉)
University of Vermont, Burlington, VT, USA
e-mail: alerellini@gmail.com

asked how likely they were to rape a woman if they could be 100 % certain they would never be caught. An alarming 35 % of respondents indicated at least some likelihood [6], confirming that we live in a culture where sexual abuse is a partially accepted.

5.1 Historical Overview of Sexual Abuse Research

In order to understand the current picture of sexual function in sexual abuse survivors, it is important to understand the history of this research. In particular, a historic overview can help us place current knowledge on sexual function of sexual abuse survivors within the larger context of mental health since sexual function has only recently joined the topics studied in the world of trauma research. The first decade of studies on sexual abuse (1960–1970) was mostly spent documenting the prevalence of sexual abuse and the high comorbidity between these traumatic experiences and negative consequences during adulthood [3]. Theoretical models and research studies initially focused on Traumatic Stress Disorder, but shortly it became clear that most, if not all, psychiatric conditions overlapped with a history of childhood sexual abuse. During these first years, very little was known about the consequences on adult sexual function outside of few clinical observations of patients that reported feeling as if they were "damaged goods" [7]. After the field was shocked by findings indicating that a third of the female population was in danger of experiencing sexual abuse and that these types of experiences were at the root of many psychiatric conditions, scholars begun to ask questions about mechanisms. The attention was now directed toward answering the question of how a sexual trauma leads to negative outcomes during adulthood. Findings from the first scattered research studies were compiled into theoretical models proposed to explain this phenomenon.

The most cited theoretical models that withheld the test of time have in common the inclusion of key developmental ages when the individual forms the skills to adapt to his or her environment and a focus on biopsychological factors that interfere with the normal processing and controlling of emotional responses [8–10]. These models challenged the idea that the sexual nature of the abuse is a key aspect and redirected our attention toward the effect that any traumatic experience may have on functioning. Research has confirmed this view; it is now well accepted that (1) sexual abuse rarely occurs alone since the norm is for multiple forms of childhood abuse (i.e., physical and emotional abuse) to co-occur [11], and (2) all forms of childhood abuse can have equally negative outcomes on adult functioning ([12, 39]). Because of these main points, it is important to carefully interpret the results from studies that list sexual abuse as the sole cause of the sexual problem and that do not report on the larger picture of the childhood of the individual. Another point that is worth noting is that the great majority of research has focused on sexual abuse during childhood. Sexual trauma, including rape, is an experience that occurs also during adolescence (after age 16) and adulthood. The negative consequences of rape have been reported in the literature, but there is a dearth of research on the sexual consequences on rape [13]. Although it may be tempting to generalize from the studies on childhood sexual abuse to a population of women sexually abused as adults (or teenagers), we should be aware that this may lead to a misunderstanding of the nature of the problems of this population [14].

Studies on sexual function in adult survivors of childhood abuse lag behind. However, over the past two decades, the coordinated efforts of a spare number of research laboratories spread throughout the globe have provided initial evidence that helps us identify a guiding model that explains how adverse childhood experiences (sexual, physical, and emotional abuse) can affect adult sexual functioning. Initial studies have also begun to tackle the question of how treatment can help these individuals to improve their sexual function or satisfaction. One area of sex research that has been neglected is male sexual abuse. It was not until recently that scholars begun to investigate sexual abuse in males and for this reason we have yet to gain a good understanding of whether the models and the evidence regarding the sexual function of adult women exposed to childhood sexual abuse can be applied to the lives of adult men. For this reason, the literature utilized for the preparation of this chapter focuses on women.

5.2 Epidemiology of Sexual Function in Survivors of Childhood Abuse

Overall, studies have identified a larger percentage of sexual dysfunction in women survivors of childhood abuse compared to women with no history of abuse [15]. However, the results are mixed, with studies using clinical samples finding double the prevalence of sexual arousal disorder, hypoactive sexual desire, and orgasmic disorder in abused women as compared to women with no history of abuse [16]. However, studies using the college population find much smaller effect sizes or no significant differences in levels of sexual function between women with and without a history of childhood sexual abuse [11, 17]. These results are confusing mostly because of the heterogeneity of individuals grouped under the "childhood abuse" label and the diverse sexual problems studied. The first discrepancy in the literature lies in the definition of sexual "problems" (for a review see [18]). Some scholars focus on problems with sexual function, including low sexual desire, difficulties with orgasm and sexual arousal, and sexual pains. On the other hand, other researchers have focused on hyperactive sexuality, including promiscuous sexual relationships, no use (or inconsistent use) of barriers during sex, and numerous sequential sexual partners. Rarely studies have focused on both sexual function and hypersexuality despite the fact that many clinical observations have reported that individuals with a history of sexual abuse may have problems in both categories: An individual may experience hypoactive sexual desire within an intimate sexual relationship but may feel sex is too frequent and out of control when not romantically involved [13].

To increase confusion on this topic, hypersexuality remains a poorly understood phenomenon. At times, the literature refers to hypersexuality as compulsive sexual behaviors, and other times as addictive sexual behaviors. Yet other research supports the conceptualization of these sexual problems as impulsive sexual behaviors [19]. Impulsivity is perhaps the concept that fits best the experience of individuals with a history of abuse. However, the scarce information available on the motivation and the precedents of these sexual behaviors prevents making a decision between compulsive, addictive, or impulsive behaviors.

5.3 Current Understanding of Sexual Dysfunction in Survivors of Childhood Abuse

The field of sexual medicine is in its infancy for what concerns the proposal and testing of a model that can explain the sexual difficulties of individuals with a history of childhood abuse. A series of studies initially conducted by Rellini and colleagues [20, 21] and confirmed by other laboratories [14] pointed to the importance of physiological and subjective impairments in the sexual responses of survivors of sexual abuse. These laboratory studies utilized vaginal photoplethysmography, a device to assess vaginal blood flow that is assessed during exposure to audio/visual erotic stimuli presented in a private room [22]. Results from this body of work showed that women with a history of childhood sexual abuse have a weaker vaginal response to sexual stimuli compared to women with no history of abuse and that this is true specifically for women with a history of childhood sexual abuse who complain about having sexual problems. Most importantly, among women who report sexual problems, those who have a history of childhood sexual abuse show a much weaker sexual response as compared to those with no history of abuse [23]. These findings corroborate that (1) a history of childhood sexual abuse does not necessarily impact the sexual function of all the survivors, and (2) those survivors who experience sexual dysfunction present a sexual response that is quite atypical even when compared to the sexual response of other women with sexual dysfunction.

To further investigate these results, scholars directed their attention to potential physiological and psychological mechanisms that could account for this weaker sexual response. A body of research specifically focused on sexual self-schemas [24–26]. Sexual self-schemas are blueprints of how people make sense of the sexual self and provide them with a map to understand their responses to sexual stimuli. Schemas are implicit and non-volitional; thus they can be activated and can function outside of consciousness. However, it is also true that we are aware of our views of ourselves; thus schemas are accessible to consciousness. Moreover, schemas can be shaped by explicit memories; thus daily experiences can shape the way the individual thinks of the self. The impact of experiences on schemas is particularly interesting to clinical scholars because through the manipulation of behaviors and memories, an individual can modify a schema. Since schemas affect physiological responses (a person's attitude about a situation dictates his/her emotional response to that situation), then scholars can affect physiological responses through the manipulation of behavior. For example, the way we think about our self affects our emotional responses and emotions are, partially, neurochemical responses that can affect blood flow, heart rate, and other physiological mechanisms influencing sexual arousal and orgasm. Thus, a modification in sexual self-schemas could affect physiological sexual responses.

Our current understanding of sexual self-schemas comes from studies on the development of scales to measure these constructs [27]. Such studies found that, although there are hundreds of ways to describe the sexual self, all sexual self-schemas can be divided roughly into three main categories: open/direct, passionate/romantic, and embarrassed/conservative (Andersen and Cyranowski). Despite this categorization being far from exhaustive, it is useful for what concerns the understanding of women with a history of sexual abuse [18].

Because schemas are both implicit and explicit, studies have utilized methodologies to tap into both these dimensions using direct and indirect measure of sexual self-schemas [24, 25]. Direct methods, such as self-reported questionnaires (i.e., Sexual Self-Schema Scale; [27]) and sexual beliefs/attitudes measures), ask directly what the individual thinks of herself as a sexual being or what are her attitudes toward different sexual matters. Romantic/passionate individuals see themselves as prone to feeling moved by situations when they feel emotionally connected with an individual. Statistical models suggest that when the sexual abuse leads to a less romantic/passionate view of the self, the individual tends to feel more negative affect during sexual activities with a partner [25]. Perhaps, in these individuals, the abuse tainted the romantic view of the self and this has led to a loss in their ability to enjoy sexual encounters. This finding makes sense in light of results from another study pointing to sexual abuse from a partner to be more strongly associated with lower sexual satisfaction than abuse perpetrated from a family member (nonparent) or acquaintance [11]. Specifically, we would expect that an abuse that occurs from a romantic partner may have a more detrimental effect on the trust of the individual in intimate relationships than an abuse coming from a non-partner.

Interestingly, the effects of schemas on sexual function are independent from symptoms of depression and anxiety [25], providing evidence that depression and anxiety are not necessary for the development of sexual problems in women who experienced sexual abuse. From this, it can be extrapolated that the individual's sexual dysfunction is not necessarily secondary to other psychiatric conditions but can emerge independently. The independence between sexual dysfunctions and other psychiatric conditions was also documented in other cross-sectional and clinical studies. For example, a study investigated sexual function, posttraumatic stress disorder symptoms, and daily stressors in a sample of adult women with a history of childhood sexual abuse recruited from the community [28]. Common sense would suggest that more severe symptoms of posttraumatic stress disorders are associated with greater sexual problems, and this was confirmed by the findings. However, more counterintuitive was the finding that daily stressors had a stronger relationship with sexual dysfunction than posttraumatic stress disorder symptoms, suggesting that clinicians should not assume that severe psychiatric conditions are the only things affecting the sexual well-being of their patients. In agreement with this finding, clinical outcome studies found that the successful treatment of depression and posttraumatic stress disorder symptoms does not automatically translate into an improvement in the sexual well-being of the individual [29–31].

A traumatic experience can affect the brain in a number of ways. One of the most intriguing and least understood mechanisms affected by trauma are perhaps the implicit processes. Our brain is wired to process a number of stimuli automatically. At any given time, we scan the world for stimuli and place such stimuli in broad categories that scholars call *appetitive* or *threatening*. Appetitive stimuli are stimuli that we are predisposed to approach. We scan the world around us and are quickly able to direct our attention to those stimuli that are appetitive and can fulfill some of our basic needs. On the other hand, we are also wired to quickly detect potentially threatening stimuli so that we can be prepared for fight or flight. Sexual stimuli are recognized as strong appetitive stimuli since they are able to capture our attention quickly and effectively. The speed with which we are able to detect stimuli has to do with the automation of our cognitive processes that allows us to scan and label stimuli. For example, scholars have found that automatic implicit associations use simple valence categories (positive or negative valence) to quickly identify important stimuli [32]. To the extent that some of these automatic associations are formed through experiences and that there are some developmental key points when these associations form more strongly, it is feasible that early negative sexual experiences may have promoted a stronger association between sex stimuli and negative valence than in other people with no negative sexual experiences. Two studies have provided initial evidence that a history of childhood sexual abuse may have rewired the brain to interpret sexual stimuli as threatening or at least as *not* appetitive. One study observed that some women with a history of childhood sexual abuse responded to sexual stimuli with an increase in the stress hormone cortisol, an indication of the activation of the stress response [21]. A second study, utilizing a behavioral measure of implicit associations (known as the Implicit Association Task: IAT, [33]), compared women with a history of sexual abuse to women with no history of abuse on the strength of the associations between sex/pleasure and neutral/pleasure [26]. For women with no history of abuse, sexual stimuli were more closely associated with pleasure than neutral stimuli, but that as not the case for the abused group for whom sex and neutral stimuli were equally associated with pleasure. These findings are particularly important in light of the fact that in neither of these studies women reported a more negative or less positive preference or liking of sexual stimuli compared to the non-abused group. Thus, clinicians should keep in mind that some of the aftermath of the sexual abuse may not be observable through measures that require self-report and that the problem, although still grounded in cognitive processes, may lay underneath the level of consciousness.

5.4 Assessment and Treatment

Clinical research has not clearly identified an efficacious treatment for the sexual dysfunction of women with a history of sexual abuse. Clinicians often recommend a complete assessment of the psychiatric difficulties of individuals with a history of sexual abuse since research shows a large overlap and co-occurrence of multiple psychiatric conditions in these individuals. Assessment should include questions to diagnose eating disorders, personality disorders (especially borderline personality disorder), mood disorders (including bipolar disorder, major depression, and dysthymia), substance abuse and dependence, and anxiety disorders (paying particular attention to posttraumatic stress disorder and phobias). The assessment of sexual dysfunction should be comprehensive and an attempt should be made to assess whether the patient feels the history of abuse has affected current functioning in any of the areas of sexual function. While completing the assessment the clinician should be careful to not assume that the abuse is the cause of dysfunction. Not all women with a history of sexual abuse develop sexual difficulties and assuming that any sexual problem can be traced back to an abusive experience may fail to understand fully the difficulty of the individual. For this reason, sexual abuse should be entertained as a causal factor only as part of a working hypothesis to share with the patient. Indeed, treating a sexual dysfunction as caused by an abuse regardless of the patient's interpretation of her problem may be perceived as invalidating of her experience and may lead to a breach in the clinician/patient relationship.

The field has not come to an agreement on the type of psychotherapy that is most appropriate for sexual dysfunctions experienced by survivors of sexual abuse. The lack of controlled clinical outcome studies does not allow for a clear suggestion on the type of approach to adopt. In general, clinicians suggest to treat any psychiatric condition (e.g., eating disorder, posttraumatic stress, depression, generalized anxiety) prior to treating the sexual dysfunction since the sexual problem could potentially be secondary to the other psychiatric conditions [34]. This approach makes sense if the person is experiencing high levels of distress caused by comorbid psychiatric conditions. However, it does not make clinician sense if the individual is coming into the clinic seeking treatment for the sexual difficulty per se. Also, from an evidence-based approach to treatment, there is very little evidence that the treatment of the comorbid psychiatric conditions alleviates the sexual problems [29–31]. A recent clinical study that utilized emotive writing and focused the attention of the patient on her sexual self-schemas showed that symptoms of depression and posttraumatic stress disorder, as well as symptoms of sexual dysfunction, improved as part of the treatment [35]. Thus, it is possible that addressing sexual self-schemas can have generalizable effects on other psychiatric symptoms. However, it is important to note the convenience sample utilized for this study which does not allow us to extrapolate any suggestions in terms of when it is appropriate to address sexual dysfunctions before (or concurrently to) other psychiatric symptoms. It is encouraging though to see positive effects on sexual function after individuals are able to demonstrate a shift in their sexual self-schemas, especially given the body of literature that supports the effects of sexual abuse on sexual self-schemas.

Another approach utilized specifically to treat sexual dysfunction that has been found particularly useful with adult women with a history of childhood sexual abuse was first tested by Brotto and colleagues [36, 37]. In her Mindfulness Based approach, Brotto teaches women to be present in the moment and paying attention to their body during sexual activities. It remains unclear why this approach is particularly useful for women with a history of childhood sexual abuse, but the results of two non-controlled trials remain positive and encouraging [36, 37]. The clinical trials have found that individuals following the treatment have greater subjective levels of sexual arousal (as measured in the laboratory) and this increases the concordance between mind and body. From these results, it can be hypothesized that, for women with a history of childhood sexual abuse who experience difficulties becoming sexually aroused, their mind is distracted and separated from their bodies during sexual activities. The treatment helps the individual to keep their mind closely connected to their bodies and this increases their sensations of sexual arousal. If this were to be true, it may be easier to understand results from a study using sildenafil showing that medication-induced increases in physiological sexual responses (i.e., vaginal blood flow) in women with a history of childhood sexual abuse resulted in a greater level of distress [38]: perhaps the greater genital sexual arousal induced by the medication widened the gap between mind and body and increased the distress experienced by these women.

References

1. Kempe CH (1977) Closing comments. Child Abuse Negl 1:511–513
2. Kempe CH (1978) Recent developments in the field of child abuse. Child Abuse Negl 2: 261–267
3. Besharov DJ (1977) U.S. National center on child abuse and neglect: three years of experience. Child Abuse Negl 1:173–177
4. Testa M, VanZile-Tamsen C, Livingston JA (2007) Prospective prediction of women's sexual victimization by intimate and non intimate male perpetrators. J Consult Clin Psychol 75:52–60
5. Öberg K, Fugl-Meyer KS, Fugl-Meyer AR (2002) On sexual well being in sexually abused Swedish women: epidemiological aspects. Sex Relation Ther 17:329–341
6. Malamuth NM (1981) Rape proclivity among males. J Soc Issues 37:138–157
7. Becker JD, Kaplanm MS (1991) Rape victims: issues, theories, and treatment. Annu Rev Sex Res 2:267–292
8. Cicchetti D, Rogosch FA, Gunnar MR, Toth SL (2010) The differential impacts of early physical and sexual abuse and internalizing problems on daytime cortisol rhythm in school-aged children. Child Dev 81:252–269
9. Finkelhor D, Browne A (1985) The traumatic impact of child sexual abuse: a conceptualization. Am J Orthopsychiatry 55:530–541
10. Linehan M (1993) Dialectical and biosocial underpinning of treatment. In: Cognitive and behavioral treatment of personality disorder. pp 28–65
11. Rellini AH, Meston CM (2007) Sexual function and satisfaction in adults based on the definition of child sexual abuse. J Sex Med 4:1312–1321

12. Seehuus MO, Clifton J, Rellini AH (in press) The role of family environment and multiple forms of childhood abuse in the shaping of sexual function and satisfaction in women. Arch Sex Behav
13. Rellini AH (2006) Psychological factors of sexual abuse on women's sexual functioning. In: Goldstein I, Meston CM, Davis SR, Traish AM (eds) Women's sexual function and dysfunction: study, diagnosis, and treatment. Taylor & Francis, New York, NY, pp 98–104
14. Schacht RL, George WH, Heiman JR, Davis KC, Norris J, Stoner SA, Kajumulo KF (2007) Effects of alcohol intoxication and instructional set on women's sexual arousal vary based on sexual abuse history. Arch Sex Behav. http://www.springerlink.com/content/9746g71568846720/fulltext.html
15. Leonard LM, Follette VM (2002) Sexual functioning in women reporting a history of child sexual abuse: review of the empirical literature and clinical implications. Annu Rev Sex Res 13:346–388
16. Loeb TB, Williams JK, Carmona JV, Rivkin I, Wyatt GE, Chin T, Asuan-O'Brien A (2002) Child sexual abuse: associations with the sexual functioning of adolescents and adults. Annu Rev Sex Res 13:307–345
17. Meston CM, Heiman JR, Trapnell PD (1999) The relation between early abuse and adult sexuality. J Sex Res 36:385–395
18. Rellini AH (2008) Review of the empirical evidence for a theoretical model to understand the sexual problems of women with a history of CSA. J Sex Med 5:31–46
19. Bancroft J, Vukadinovic Z (2004) Sexual addiction, sexual compulsivity, sexual impulsivity, or what? Toward a theoretical model. J Sex Res 41:225–234
20. Rellini AH, Meston CM (2006) Psychophysiological sexual arousal in women with a history of child sexual abuse. J Sex Marital Ther 32:5–22
21. Rellini AH, Hamilton LD, Delville Y, Meston CM (2009) The cortisol response during physiological sexual arousal in women with a history of childhood sexual abuse. J Trauma Stress 22:557–565
22. Geer JH (2005) Development of the vaginal photoplethysmograph. Int J Impot Res 17:285–287
23. Rellini AH (2007) The sexual responses of women with a history of sexual abuse. Unpublished Dissertation, University of Texas at Austin, Austin, Texas. http://www.lib.utexas.edu/etd/d/2007/rellinia62970/rellinia62970.pdf
24. Meston CM, Rellini AH, Heiman J (2006) Women's history of sexual abuse, their sexuality, and sexual self-schemas. J Consult Clin Psychol 74:229–236
25. Rellini AH, Meston CM (2011) Sexual self-schemas, sexual dysfunction, and the sexual responses of women with a history of childhood sexual abuse. Arch Sex Behav 40:351–362
26. Rellini AH, Ing AD, Meston CM (2011) Implicit and explicit cognitive sexual processes in survivors of childhood sexual abuse. J Sex Med 8:3098–3107
27. Andersen BL, Cyranowski JM (1994) Women's sexual self-schema. J Pers Soc Psychol 67(6):1079
28. Zollman G, Rellini AH, Desrocher D (2013) The mediating effect of daily stress on the sexual arousal function of women with a history of childhood sexual abuse. J Sex Marital Ther 39:176–192
29. Rieckert J, Möller AT (2000) Rational-emotive behavior therapy in the treatment of adult victims of childhood sexual abuse. J Ration Emotion Cogn Behav Ther 18:87–101
30. Follette VM (1991) Marital therapy for sexual abuse survivors. New Dir Ment Health Serv 91:61–71
31. Classen CC, Palesh OG, Cavanaugh CE, Koopman C, Kaupp JW, Kraemer HC, Aggarwal R, Spiegel D (2011) A comparison of trauma-focused and present-focused group therapy for survivors of childhood sexual abuse: a randomized controlled trial. Psychol Trauma 3:84–93
32. Klinger MR, Greenwald AG (1995) Unconscious priming of association judgments. J Exp Psychol Learn Mem Cogn 21:569–581

33. Greenwald AG, McGhee DE, Schwartz JLK (1998) Measuring individual differences in implicit cognition: the Implicit Association Test. J Pers Soc Psychol 74:1464–1480
34. Maltz W (2002) Treating the sexual intimacy concerns of sexual abuse survivors. Sex Relation Ther 17:321–327
35. Meston CM, Lorenz TA, Stephenson KR (2013) Effects of expressive writing on sexual dysfunction, depression, and PTSD in women with a history of childhood sexual abuse: results from a randomized clinical trial. J Sex Med 10:2177–2189
36. Brotto LA, Basson R, Luria M (2008) A mindfulness-based group psychoeducational intervention targeting sexual arousal disorder in women. J Sex Med 5:1646–1659
37. Brotto LA, Seal BN, Rellini AH (2012) Pilot study of a brief cognitive behavioral versus mindfulness-based intervention for women with sexual distress and a history of childhood sexual abuse. J Sex Marital Ther 38:1–27
38. Berman LA, Berman JR, Bruck D, Pawar RV, Goldstein I (2001) Pharmacotherapy or psychotherapy? Effective treatment for FSD related to unresolved childhood sexual abuse. J Sex Marital Ther 27:421–425
39. Schloredt KA, Heiman JR (2003) Perceptions of sexuality as related to sexual functioning and sexual risk in women with different types of childhood abuse histories. J Trauma Stress 16:275–284

Childhood Sexual Abuse and Psychopathology

Giovanni Castellini, Mario Maggi, and Valdo Ricca

6.1 Definition and Methodological Issues

The role of negative, unfortunate events in the causation of mental disorders has always been deeply rooted in popular beliefs as well as in the history of psychiatry. Early life events are those occurring during childhood/adolescence and have a role of predisposing factor for many psychiatric conditions. Research over the last 30 years has established a significant relationship between childhood sexual abuse (CSA)—defined as a sexual encounter in which touching or penetration of the genitals happened before age 16 with someone at least 5 years older [1]—and a range of mental health and behavioral problems in adult life [2]. Meta-analyses, systematic reviews, and even reviews of reviews attempted to summarize the huge number of empirical studies on the relationship between history of CSA and psychopathology, and they generally found a significant association with a lifetime diagnosis of personality disorders (especially with borderline personality disorder), anxiety disorders (especially with posttraumatic stress disorder, panic disorder, agoraphobia, and obsessive–compulsive disorder), mood disorders (especially

---

G. Castellini
Department of Experimental, Clinical and Biomedical Sciences, University of Florence, Viale Pieraccini, 6, Florence 50134, Italy

Department of Neuropsychiatric Sciences, University of Florence, Largo Brambilla 3, Florence 50134, Italy
e-mail: giovannicastellini78@hotmail.com

M. Maggi
Department of Experimental, Clinical and Biomedical Sciences, University of Florence, Viale Pieraccini, 6, Florence 50134, Italy
e-mail: mario.maggi@unifi.it

V. Ricca (✉)
Department of Neuropsychiatric Sciences, University of Florence, Largo Brambilla 3, Florence 50134, Italy
e-mail: valdo.ricca@unifi.it

major depression and bipolar illness), disruptive behavior disorders, eating disorders, dissociative disorders, sleep disorders, and suicide attempts [3–6]. On the other hand, less clear relationship is reported with schizophrenia or somatoform disorders. Apart from the nature of the disorder taken into account, what results to be clear from the meta-analytic approach is the relevant heterogeneity of the findings considering the relationship between CSA and specific diagnoses. There are several reasons for this heterogeneity, which we attempted to summarize in this section.

First of all, **methodological issues** probably contribute to inconsistent findings within studies. Most of them used predominately cross-sectional designs based on case–control approach. Cases are usually taken from clinical settings but with control samples drawn from settings ranging from psychiatric clinics to primary care and population-based samples [3, 7, 8]. Stronger associations were generally reported when the control group was nonclinical as opposed to findings of no difference when the control group consisted of clinical patients, particularly those with other psychopathological features [3, 8]. Nevertheless, evidence of greater reliability and generalizability can be derived from studies utilizing large random community samples, birth cohorts, and twin cohorts. Moreover, the retrospective design may bias the assessment of early events in several ways. It is based on the assumption that there is a close correspondence between the history of abuse given in adult life and the actual events in childhood. However, retrospective evaluations of adverse experiences in childhood could be influenced by current adulthood psychopathology. The poor reliability of the memories relevant to childhood [9, 10] could be the consequence of the "search for meaning," by which the subjects tend to search the reasons for the present distress in their past experiences, the attitude of the interviewer, who may or may not encourage the patient, all possibly able to affect the accurate retrieval of past events [11]. On the other side, recollections of past stressful experiences could be influenced by memory distortions such as dissociative amnesia or denial, which could result in underreporting [12]. Therefore, the most reliable way to assess childhood trauma is to externally corroborate it, which is quite difficult in an experimental setting.

It is important to note that the term risk factor is currently defined as an "influence that predates the onset of the disorder and increases the likelihood that the disorder will develop" [5]. Therefore, only longitudinal, prospective research can definitively establish the required temporal relationship, and they allow to clarify causal priority, control of confounding variables, avoidance of recall, and sampling bias. However, although methodologically superior, they face the hurdle of how to obtain follow-up data on the abused children and show ethical (e.g., researcher reporting abuse) and practical (e.g., excessive costs, long time, and associated attrition) issues [13].

An example of reliable representative investigation on CSA is the Cutajar et al. [13] study, which involved almost 3,000 children whose sexual abuse was investigated at the time by forensic medical examinations. Child sexual abuse cases were identified using the records of the Victorian Institute of Forensic Medicine (VIFM), which since 1957 has provided medical examinations in cases of suspected

CSA. Subsequent psychopathology was established using a database which provides comprehensive coverage of all contacts and treatment episodes with the public mental health services in Victoria (Australia). This study, overcoming many of the limitations of previous studies, found that victims of CSA suffered three times the burden of mental health problems (in both childhood and adulthood) compared to members of the general community. Another investigation which may be mentioned as a good example of reliable study is that performed by Jonas et al. [14] which used the detailed information available from the 2007 Adult Psychiatric Morbidity Survey of England (APMS 2007) in order to quantify links between CSA and a range of psychiatric conditions. It was based on a large random sample of the English household population and used standardized methods to establish the diagnosis of specific psychiatric conditions. Of all the six types of common mental disorder investigated (depressive episode, mixed anxiety/depressive disorder, generalized anxiety disorder, panic disorder, phobic disorder, and obsessive–compulsive disorder), as well as alcohol abuse and drug abuse, posttraumatic stress disorder and eating disorders were found to be strongly and highly significantly associated with CSA.

According to an overview of meta-analyses on CSA, it is noteworthy the apparent lack of **specificity** of CSA for any diagnostic category. CSA has been found to be a possible risk factor even for different medical conditions such as chronic medical conditions [15], and sexual abuse survivors make up a sizable percentage (estimated at 13–26 %) of primary care practices [5]. The lack of diagnostic specificity seems to be common in psychiatry. Moreover, having one single diagnosis is unusual in psychiatry, where comorbidity is the rule [16]. It would be more logical to reverse the course of the research process: first to clarify an abnormality among the broad spectrum of psychiatric disorders and then to explore the clinical aspects (including the diagnosis) that are related to such abnormality. On the other hand, considering that the various forms of childhood abuse may have different developmental effects, researchers have emphasized the need to examine the various forms of abuse separately [17, 18]. However, it should be noted at the outset that comorbidity among abuse types is common [19], which makes our effort to find specific effects for individual forms of abuse more difficult.

In conclusion, since CSA is a risk factor for many forms of psychopathology and hence tells us little about the development of a disorder per se, the specificity of CSA for different psychiatric diagnosis seems to be poor. The commonly recognized multifactorial models for mental illness are based on the assumption that almost all psychiatric conditions are caused by a sequence or combination of risk factors rather than a single influence. Accordingly, CSA may combine with certain other risk factors to result in a specific diagnosis, while combining with others can lead to other psychopathological outcomes. In other words, different **moderators** and **mediators** may affect the extent and nature of the relationship between CSA and psychopathology. If each form of abuse is related to a variety of psychopathology, then the research should focus on the moderators, or factors that may make the development of one disorder versus another more likely. Once that the relationship has been proved, the research should focus on the mediators which

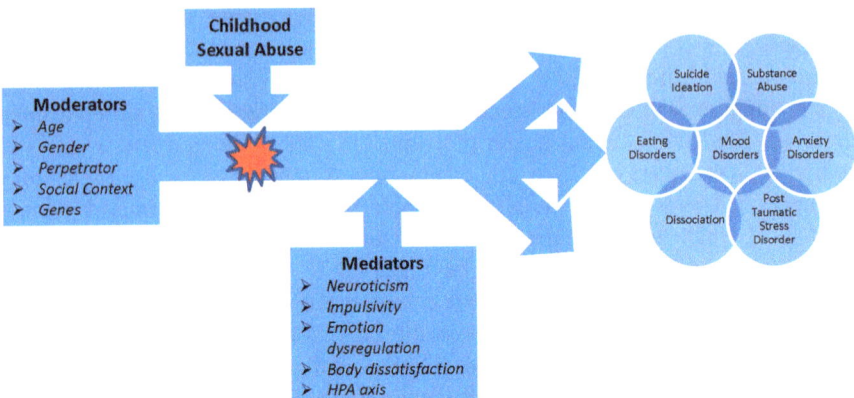

Fig. 6.1 Moderators and Mediators of Psychopathology development in subjects reporting Childhood Sexual Abuse

explain the generative mechanism through which CSA is able to influence the development of later psychopathology. Figure 6.1 reports an explicative model of the role of moderators and mediators variables in the relationship between CSA and psychopathology.

6.2 Childhood Sexual Abuse and Specific Psychopathological Outcomes

It is plausible that a traumatic event, such as CSA, occurring in crucial period for developing social relationship, emotion regulation process, mature self-representation and therefore personality, may result in severe personality disorders in adolescent and adulthood. Cutajar et al.'s study [13] provides strong confirmatory evidence for CSA being a risk factor for developing severe personality disorders. According to other studies in this [20, 21], **borderline personality disorder** (BPD) was found seven times more often among female victims. On the contrary, male victims developed antisocial personality disorder significantly more often, instead of showing an excess of borderline diagnosis. Authors hypothesized that the difference was due to the males' tendency to externalize their distress, or perhaps to the diagnostic prejudices of mental health professionals. Some scholars supported the model that severe personality disorders such as BPD are related to sexual, physical, and emotional abuse, and severe neglect by primary caretakers [22, 23], rather than to other early life events such as separations or loss [24]. On the contrary, the development of depression would be predisposed by different early life events, such as those involving loss, death, or separation, especially when the depression is severe [25]. However, several behaviours and pathological features of BPD which are commonly associated with a history of CSA are widespread in a plethora of different psychopathological conditions. Examples are impulsive behaviours which are frequently associated with eating disorders, or dissociation, or self-harm. The same BPD is often comorbid with mood, anxiety, and eating disorders.

Indeed, CSA appears to be an important risk factor also for depressive and anxiety disorders in adulthood, particularly in cases of comorbid depression and anxiety [26]. Community-based studies on children, youth, and adult populations have consistently found a moderate or strong relationship between **depressive symptoms** and reported history of CSA [13, 27, 28], with meta-analyses revealing odds ratios for reported CSA history ranging from 2.1 to 7.0 times greater among those with depression [29]. Cutajar et al. [13] found that the affective disorders, mainly major depression, were found twice as often as expected, which falls at the lower level of reported ratios [29, 30]. Finally, CSA was found to be a strong predictor of long-term trajectory and outcome of Dysthymic disorder [31]. As a possible mechanism, it has been postulated that CSA may alter the child's belief system and subsequently contribute to the development of cognitive vulnerability, in particular learned helplessness and an external locus of control [2].

As far as anxiety disorders are concerned, a meta-analysis reported CSA was 1.3–4.3 times greater in subjects suffering from an **anxiety disorder** [32]. Although many population and clinical studies on youth and adults support a strong relationship between retrospectively reported CSA and **posttraumatic stress disorder** (PTSD), few community studies have examined the relationship with other anxiety disorders [33]. Cutajar et al. [13] study found that anxiety disorders were twice the expected level in the general population and that these conditions were comorbid with **drug** and **alcohol abuse** in subjects who reported CSA.

There is a widely held clinical view that persons with histories of sexual abuse in childhood not only have higher rates of disorders such as depression or anxiety, but are more prone to have multiple problems [13, 34] including substance abuse and suicide. In general, childhood traumata were associated with an earlier age of onset of alcohol and other substance abuse [35]. Other population-based studies found higher frequencies of history of CSA among adolescents and adults with alcohol- and/or drug-related disorders compared to non-abused counterparts, with odds ratios ranging from 1.01 to 8.9 [13, 27, 29, 36].

A family study of childhood maltreatment including 2,559 subjects [37] found that a history of CSA was associated with increased risk of major depression and particularly **suicidal thoughts** and behaviour including suicidal ideation, persistent suicidal thoughts, suicide plan, and suicide attempt (both lifetime and recurrent). CSA was found to be associated with increased risk of suicidal ideation [38] and suicide attempt [39, 40]. As a matter of fact, suicide behaviour is not associated only with mood disorders, and therefore the association between CSA and suicide appeared to be trans-nosographic. For example, a strong association of CSA with suicidal behaviour has been reported in college students [41] and psychosomatic clinic patients [39] of both genders. In the Christchurch Health and Development Study [29], a longitudinal study in a population representative adolescent sample, significant CSA-associated risk of suicidal ideation and suicide attempt was found for both young men and women.

A large number of studies have been focused on the relationship between CSA and **eating disorders** (EDs). CSA has been suggested as an important but nonspecific risk factor for the development of ED symptoms. Elevated rates of child abuse have consistently been identified in ED samples [42, 43], and a recent meta-analysis [3] showed that they are particularly associated with a diagnosis of Bulimia Nervosa. This field of research is particularly affected by the methodological issues raised above. Indeed recent reviews showed that CSA is a nonspecific retrospective correlate of anorexia and bulimia nervosa [42] and a risk factor for bulimia nervosa with significant comorbidity [7]. As stated in the previous paragraph, to confirm CSA as a risk factor for ED longitudinal studies are needed. Johnson et al.'s [44] study was one of the few truly longitudinal investigations on the relationship between CSA and EDs. Childhood abuse was ascertained by reports to a child protection registry and by maternal interview. Johnson et al. found that CSA was a risk factor for EDs in early adulthood in a community sample of 782 mothers and their offspring. Offspring were interviewed at the ages of 6, 14, 16, and 22 years, but there was temporal overlap between assessment of CSA and eating disorder in the adolescent age group, making the directional nature of the association between CSA and eating disorder unclear. Another reliable survey was the one by Sanci et al. [8], based on the Victorian Adolescent Health Cohort Study. This study provides evidence that CSA is a risk factor for bulimic disorders in young females. It showed also the additive effect of reiterative CSA, as Sanci et al. found that reporting 2 or more episodes of CSA before the age of 16 years predicted a greater than fivefold elevated cumulative risk of new bulimic syndrome during adolescence. Their results augment evidence reported by the review of Jacobi et al. [42] who found that in four of the five eligible studies higher rates of CSA were present for patients with bulimia and anorexia nervosa, but that the evidence was much stronger for bulimia nervosa. Several alternative explanations have been posed for the development of eating disorders among women with a history of childhood sexual abuse. Sexual abuse may act specifically by inducing feelings of poor self-esteem, which could trigger self-starvation, as a reflection of the individual's effort at regaining control on her life [3]. Alternatively, sexual victimization may lead a woman to feel revulsion about her body in a way that may manifest with concerns about body weight, shape, and size. Details of the putative mechanism which related CSA to specific psychopathology are discussed in the next two sections more in depth.

The relationship between CSA and EDs has been often considered to be mediated by **dissociation** [45], which consists in "a disruption in the usually integrated functions of consciousness, memory, identity, and perception of the environment" [46]. Dissociation plays an important role in binge eating severity for subjects with bulimic symptoms [45] and it is partially involved in the most well-documented theories about binge eating: the "mood modulation" theory [47] and the "escape" theory [48]. However, dissociation is not always associated with EDs, but it is widespread across several different psychiatric conditions, such as PTSD, somatoform disorders, and the dissociative identity disorder which constitutes the extreme form of dissociation. Dissociation may begin either suddenly or gradually and may be transient or chronic. From a clinical point of view, five different symptom groups should be considered: amnesia, de-personalization, de-realization, mixed identity, and identity fragmentation. In general, dissociative disorder has been found resulting from long-lasting early-onset childhood trauma [12, 49] even if some authors argued that not all dissociative experiences are associated with a history of trauma. It is not clear which aspects of childhood maltreatment influence the development and nature of trauma-related dissociative symptoms. However, dissociation related to trauma may involve disruptions or breakdowns of memory, awareness, identity, and/or perception ("psychoform dissociation") as well as losses or distortion of sensory, perceptual, affective, or motor functions ("somatoform dissociation"; [50]). In particular, epidemiological studies of nonclinical samples [51] and psychiatric populations [52] found that childhood maltreatment before the age of 13 years represents a risk factor for development of severe dissociation in adulthood.

Overall, the large number of studies performed in the last 10 years about the effects of childhood trauma in adulthood confirmed a lack of specific interrelationships between CSA and psychopathology, supporting the hypothesis of general vulnerability for psychopathology among individuals exposed to early childhood trauma. Moreover, these findings challenge the approach based on categorical mental disorder diagnoses and support those studies aimed at the investigation of CSA as a potential risk factor for the development of psychological dimensions, or pathological behaviors. For instance, CSA may lead to impulsive traits which correlates with suicide, self-harm, and binge eating. Moreover, body image disturbance, which has been reported as a common outcome of sexual abuse, is a core feature of EDs, Body Dysmorphic Disorder, as well as Sexual Disorders.

6.3 Moderators of Psychopathological Outcomes of CSA

It is well known that not all traumatized children develop psychiatric symptoms. Survivors of CSA are at increased risk for developing depressive, anxiety, or eating disorders, but childhood victimization alone is not sufficient to cause these conditions. Other factors, such as severity of abuse, numbers of perpetrators, family environment, gender, age of the victim, and his/her cognitive and affect modulation capacities, may moderate the relationship between CSA and psychopathology.

Therefore, the issue of specificity of CSA long-lasting effects can be formulated by means of two research questions:
1. Is a CSA sufficient to determine a specific psychopathological outcome in adulthood?
2. Which person is more vulnerable to CSA effect?

Moderator analyses allowed to find answers to these questions. In the psychological literature, moderators represent those factors that may make the development of one disorder versus another more likely. Moreover, moderator analyses allowed to identify specific subpopulation of subjects in which a certain relationship (e.g., between CSA and psychopathology) is stronger than in the general population. According to Baron and Kenny's definition, a moderator is a qualitative or quantitative variable that affects the direction and strength of the relation between an independent (predictor variable) and a dependent variable. Furthermore, the moderator partitions a focal independent variable into subgroups that establish its domains of maximal effectiveness in regard to a given dependent variable [53]. Research of moderators is particularly important since it provides information regarding the etiology of specific conditions, even if it is multifactorial.

Age of abuse may represent an example of moderator, as it is possible that the effect of a sexual abuse differs by age. In other words, childhood developmental stage at which the maltreatment occurred would have a different association with a further development of dissociation, posttraumatic stress symptoms, depression, or eating disorder symptoms in adulthood. Even if the developmental timing of exposure to CSA is considered an important dimension that may be related to subsequent psychopathology risk [54, 55], there is little consensus on whether earlier or later exposure is associated with worse outcomes. CSA in early age is supposed to be more deleterious than later episodes because it happens during specific developmental stages, thus compromising a child's ability to successfully master stage-salient developmental tasks, including secure attachments, self-regulation, stress response, executive functioning, and arousal [55, 56]. Moreover, the damage of an early CSA may also be more severe because it occurs when the foundation of brain architecture is being wired and it can disrupt the development of neural circuits that interfere with typical patterns of brain development, heightening vulnerability to psychopathology. The neurobiological systems involved are related with regulating arousal, emotion, stress responses, and reward processing [57]. Nevertheless, it has been argued that CSA occurring in later stages might be more harmful because the person has already developed the ability to conceptualize experiences of abuse [58]. According to other studies [59, 60], Cutajar et al. [13] did not confirm that CSA in early developmental stages leads to a more severe psychiatric disability, hypothesizing that older victims, especially those undergoing sexual development, would have greater awareness of the gross violations of sexual boundaries. However, other results seem to suggest that early CSA may result not just in a more severe disability, rather in specific disorders with a more pervasive nature than others. For example, Dunn et al. [55] found that among those subjects who experienced maltreatment, a first exposure during the early childhood period, particularly during preschool (ages 3–5), would determine more deleterious effects in terms of depression and suicidal ideation in young adulthood. Furthermore, our unpublished data seem to suggest that the association between CSA and eating disorders is less significant for those who experienced the abuse over 13 years (Faravelli et al. unpublished data). Finally, Mueller-Pfeiffer et al. [12] found that psychoform dissociation was significantly related to childhood maltreatment before the age of 13 years.

As far as the moderating role of **gender** is concerned, the association between CSA and psychopathology appears to be stronger for women than men [61]. Epidemiologic data suggest that CSA-associated risks for psychiatric disorders may be less wide ranging in men. Bedi et al. [37] found evidence that women with a history of CSA attempted suicide on average more than 5 years earlier than men with a similar history. Moreover, a significant association between CSA and alcohol abuse has been observed primarily in women [62]. Finally, Cutahjar et al. [13] found a relationship between CSA and affective disorder only for female victims. These results can be explained by a true gender difference in response to abuse: for example, it has been suggested that gender differences in depression are partly explained by females' higher likelihood of experiencing interpersonal violence [55]. Alternatively, it is possible that the different pattern of association could be due to a greater tendency of females to express their distress in terms of recognizable depression by clinicians [13]. However, the literature on gender differences remains somewhat difficult to interpret, given the lower prevalence of CSA in men.

In the last 10 years the theoretical models of CSA have become more complex not just for the inclusion of variables associated with the victim (e.g., age, gender), but also because the role of the **perpetrator**'s characteristics, as well as the importance of the **social context** of the child, has been emphasized. First of all, it is possible that the perpetrator's relationship to the victim of CSA influences the development of adult psychopathology or at least the referral to a psychiatric service. Cutajar et al. [13] found that the perpetrator and characteristics of the violence were associated with diagnosis of psychopathological consequences. Indeed, CSA by multiple offenders was most strongly associated with the victim having contact with public mental health services and receiving a clinical diagnosis, while penetrative abuse was associated with a shorter time period between exposure to CSA and contact with mental health services and receiving a clinical diagnosis. An important limitation which should be considered is that a closer relationship with the perpetrator might lead to reluctance to report and a decreased memory of the sexual abuse [63]. Moreover it has been suggested that intra-familial sexual abuse may be associated with specific psychopathological conditions, such as dissociative identity disorder, which is thought to emerge in children who are faced with unresolvable dilemmas when they desire love and nurturing from frightening and neglecting attachment figures [64].

Social support has been hypothesized to be one of the protective factors that buffer children from the impact of these negative early experiences [65, 66]. Therefore, the psychopathological outcome of CSA may be influenced by characteristics of the **family** or **social support**, which allow the victim to cope with the trauma [67]. Cohen and Hoberman [68] postulate that high levels of social support protect individuals from stress-induced pathology. Social support moderates the consequences of child maltreatment, respective to depression, anxiety, and substance abuse being the most common. Perspective studies found that social support moderated the risk of affective disorders, but not substance abuse or anxiety disorders [69]. Regarding the type of social support, self-esteem and appraisal support were found to buffer against the development of PTSD in sexually abused women, while tangible and belonging support had little influence [70]. From an opposite perspective, it is important to consider the effect of CSA on development of social relationship and social environment. Accordingly, the "deterioration model" [66, 71] is based on the hypothesis that CSA exhausts social support because it elicits confusion, helplessness, and aversion in others in the long term.

A related issue is whether victims of CSA experience additional stressors, including separation from their parents, foster care placement, and multiple forms of revictimization over the course of their lives [72]. The context of abuse should be taken into account considering the frequent overlap and coexistence of adverse childhood life events and childhood trauma [73]. In general, models for CSA and psychopathology should consider the synergistic effects of CSA and different traumatic experience. For example, CSA is significantly related to later [14, 74] **revictimization**, which is defined as repetition of childhood contact abuse in adulthood. Revictimization is associated with an increased frequency of psychiatric [14]. Moreover, Favaro et al. [75] took into consideration traumas preceding the CSA, demonstrating a synergistic effect of neonatal dysmaturity and childhood abuse in increasing the risk for AN, which might be explained by the hypothesis that a prenatal programming of stress response systems can result in an impairment of the individual's resilience to severe stressful events.

The neuroscience perspective stressed the importance of taking into account a biological underpinning as a further moderator for the relationship between CSA and psychopathology. In terms of moderator analyses, this means to consider factors preceding the traumatic event, and therefore biological mechanisms accounting for an individual vulnerability to CSA effects on psychopathological outcomes. According to the **gene–environment** interaction, CSA may potentiate the development of psychiatric disorders in genetically vulnerable individuals, resulting in a reduced ability to respond to stress. Within candidate genes, the serotonin transporter gene has been the focus of several researches because of its association with depression. The New Zealand birth cohort study by Caspi et al. [76] demonstrated that people homozygous for the short form of the serotonin transporter gene promoter region polymorphism (5HTTLPR) are at higher risk of depression than people with other genotypes if they experience childhood maltreatment. The study also demonstrated that people homozygous for the long form of 5HTTLPR who have a history of childhood maltreatment are at lower risk of developing depression than people with other genotypes. This result was replicated by other studies by Kendler et al. [77] and Kaufman et al. [78] on childhood maltreatment in general, and more specifically in CSA [79]. Considering a specific association with eating disorders, it has been demonstrated that bulimic women with a history of CSA, carrying low-function alleles of the serotonin transporter promoter polymorphism, 5HTTLPR, also evince more pronounced manifestations of such traits as sensation seeking, affective instability [80], and dissocial behaviour [81].

Other scholars focused on gene–environment interaction involving the **hypothalamic–pituitary–adrenal axis** (HPA), which has been reported to increase the likelihood of development of several psychiatric disorders such as depression, PTSD, or eating disorders. Genetic effect would impact the sensitivity of HPA axis mechanisms implicated in stress responsiveness. The BcII restriction fragment length polymorphism is the most widely studied of polymorphisms associated with glucocorticoid receptor expression. This polymorphism is considered a moderator of stress-induced effects, since it is believed to modulate inhibitory feedback within the HPA axis and, in this fashion, to contribute to variability in stress reactivity [82, 83]. Steiger et al. [84] proposed an example of gene (moderator)–environment (CSA) interaction for BclI in eating disorders patients: the risk of having Bulimia Nervosa was found to be associated with the combined presence of two factors having a genetic propensity (associated with the low-function allele of the BcII polymorphism) toward lesser modulation of stress reactivity, and being exposed, in childhood, to severe physical or sexual abuse. Moreover, genetic variants in the corticotropin-releasing hormone receptor (CRHR1) gene polymorphisms were found to both predict and protect for the development of depression in persons with a history of trauma [85]. Moreover the FK506 binding protein (FKBP5) polymorphisms have been found to be associated with PTSD symptoms in adult patients with a history of childhood abuse, even if CRHR1 polymorphisms were not found to be associated with PTSD in the same population [86].

6.4 Mediators of the Relationship Between CSA and Psychopathology

Once that a specific relationship between CSA and mental symptoms has been established, research should take into account the generative mechanism through which CSA is able to influence development of later psychopathology. According to Baron and Kenny definition's [53], a given variable may be said to function as a mediator to the extent that it accounts for the relation between the predictor (CSA) and the criterion (psychopathology).

There are several conditions in which the relationship between CSA severity and specific psychopathology of interest has been found to be mediated by a third factor. **Neuroticism**—defined as propensity for negative emotionality, including anxiety, anger, hostility, and depression—has been found to mediate the relationship between sexual abuse severity and depression [87]. Neuroticism is a trait developed in childhood, sensitive to traumatic life experiences [88], which remains stable in adulthood.

A research question which could find an answer in mediator analyses is: "Why CSA is associated with suicidal thoughts?" However, the answer could be less simple than expected. For example, it is possible that the mediator is not one but more variables able to contribute to the development of different psychopathological outcomes. Clinicians usually think that relationship with suicide is mediated by depressive symptoms. In other words, victims of CSA have suicide ideation because they experience a severe form of depression. Martin et al. [89] found that in girls, depression completely mediated the association between CSA and suicidality, while Sigfusdottir et al. [90] found that, although depressed mood associated with CSA is a partial mediator and strong predictor for suicidal behavior, an association remained between CSA and suicidal behavior in adolescents not suffering from feelings of depression. Therefore, it is possible that the relationship between CSA and suicide is not mediated only by depressive symptoms but also by the development of **impulsive traits**, which account for suicide attempts, conduct disorder, or substance abuse. Impulsivity has been associated with both suicidal behaviours and borderline personality disorder [91]. CSA could interact with existing temperament (impulsivity), leading to persistent psychobiological abnormalities which impair adaptive responses to stress [92]. Impulsive suicidal patterns—emerging in specific groups of subjects (e.g., borderline personality disorder subjects)—would result from a complex interaction between temperament vulnerability and traumatic experiences.

Among the several suggested mechanisms for the association of CSA and impulsive behaviours, **emotion dysregulation** is one of the most investigated. Self-harm, suicide attempts, and eating disorder behaviours (including binge eating, purging, or starving) have been proposed as dysfunctional coping strategies to regulate the continuing emotional distress following the experience of abuse [7]. The construct of emotion regulation encompasses not just the experience of a negative mood itself, but also the ability to adaptively identify and cope with negative mood states [93]. Deficit in emotion regulation may be due not only to the CSA effects but also to other types of abuse. Indeed, more comprehensive models for psychopathology development should consider that research has shown that emotional, physical, and sexual abuse tends to coexist. Emotional maltreatment includes caregiver criticism of emotional expression, punishment of emotional expression, or minimization of emotion. All these conditions, related to emotionally abusive environments, are associated with emotional suppression, avoidant coping, and failure to seek support in children, all of which may be conceptualized as maladaptive emotion regulation strategies [93]. In adults, childhood emotional abuse has been linked to emotional inhibition and avoidant coping [94], emotional non-acceptance, and experiential avoidance [95]. According to Bowlby theory [96], emotional maltreatment by a caregiver is responsible for the development of insecure attachment styles, and insecure attachment in infancy has been linked with poor emotional regulation and social functioning in humans as well as in animal models. These effects are carried forward into adulthood, and they increase the risk of psychopathology throughout the life span. The consequences of a CSA for a child growing up in an emotionally abusive environment have several potential links to the emotion regulation model of the development of psychiatric symptoms. In general, an abusive family environment is characterized by different types of childhood adversity. It has been demonstrated that the increasing number of childhood adversities was associated with greater adult clinical complexity in terms of psychiatric comorbidities and the presence of coexisting internalizing and externalizing disorders [97]. On the contrary, an emotionally adequate family environment may act in a protective way toward CSA effects. For example, Sperry and Widom [66] found that the presence of good family and social support mediated the relationship between child maltreatment, anxiety, and depression. Indeed, they found that total social support and belonging support reduced the direct effect of child abuse/neglect on these symptoms to non-significance.

As far as specific disorders are concerned, emotion dysregulation hypothesis for the development of eating disorders symptoms proposes that symptoms such as binge eating are initiated in an effort to distract oneself from negative emotions or self-soothe [48]. In this model, disordered eating behaviours are conceptualized as a maladaptive means of dealing with negative affect, thus implying poor emotion regulation skills. Binge eating behaviour likely acts as a negative reinforcer via this pathway because it acts to decrease or block negative affect, at least in the short term, by relieving the experience of painful emotions [98]. Alternatively, bulimic symptoms have been linked to CSA by means of the mediation of dissociative symptoms. Indeed, bulimia has been viewed as a dissociative state in which awareness of CSA trauma is diminished [7, 8]; the binge/purge cycles might function as an expression of anger or a symbolic "cleansing" of the self of the abusive experience, thereby allowing an individual to regain a stronger sense of self. In line with "escape theory" by Heatherton and Baumeister's [48] negative affect induced by CSA memories and images begins the motivation to escape, which occurs by the patient narrowing his or her awareness from abstract levels (self-evaluation) to the level of the physical surroundings or stimulus. The temporary loss of inhibition results in the release of previously suppressed behaviours, such as binge eating.

A new frontier of CSA research focused on the role of **body image** and **body dissatisfaction** as potential mediators of the relationship between CSA and adult development of overlapping conditions such as eating and sexual disorders, obsessive–compulsive symptoms, and self-harm behaviours. Among victims of sexual abuse, the relationship with one's own body may be particularly affected, and CSA has a significant and lasting effect on body image and identity, as well as with self-regulation mechanisms [99]. Indeed, women with history of sexual abuse reported more body dissatisfaction [100]. It is well known that body image distortion and body uneasiness are one the core psychopathological features of eating disorders, and they represent the onset and maintaining factors for pathological eating behaviours. Preti et al. [99] found that body dissatisfaction acts as an intervening variable in the link between sexual abuse before 12 years old and eating disorder symptoms, and therefore it might be considered as a mediator in the pathways from sexual abuse to pathological eating behaviours. The complex relationship between CSA, eating disorders, and body dissatisfaction represent also an explaining model for other psychiatric symptoms, such as self-harm behaviours. Eating disorder patients with a history of abuse were found to be more likely to engage in self-destructive behaviour [75]. The recourse to self-harming behaviour in these patients has been interpreted as a way to regain control on a compromised interoceptive awareness by cutting and burning the body [99]. Compulsive cleaning behaviours have also been associated with a history of CSA by the mediation of a disease related to once own body, and specific compulsive behaviours could be interpreted as an attempt to symbolically clean out the body of the impurity associated with the past abuse [100].

Body dissatisfaction is an overlapping area of interest between CSA, eating disorder, and **sexual dysfunction**. A profound uneasiness toward once own body consequent to CSA might be the explaining mechanism also for the relationship between CSA and sexual dysfunction. Women who felt more negatively about their bodies reported lower levels of desire and sexual arousal functioning [101, 102], engaged in more sexual avoidance [103], and reported less pleasure, orgasm, and sexual satisfaction [104], as compared with women who had a more positive perception of their bodies. Sexual functioning in eating disorders patients has been associated with concerns about body image (e.g., dissatisfaction with body parts, concerns with body size or weight, discomfort with one's body in front of a partner, or others) [105]. Additionally, recent studies suggest a mediating effect of sexual dysfunction in the relationship between CSA and dangerous sexual behaviours [106].

HPA axis is the most promising candidate as biological underpinning for the relationship between CSA and psychopathology. As already stated, the glucocorticoid receptor polymorphisms have been considerate as potential moderators of the interaction. Accordingly, the effect of CSA for psychopathology during adulthood is believed to be mediated by the HPA axis that, once over-activated during the developmental processes, would remain permanently unstable, overdriven, vulnerable, or dysfunctional [11], possibly due to transcriptional/epigenomic mechanisms [11]. Indeed, early life events influence the HPA axis response during adulthood psychopathology [107]. Newport et al. [108] found that depressed women with a history of child abuse showed hyper-suppression (i.e., lower cortisol) at the response to the Dexamethasone Suppression Test (DST). Similar findings were reported for men with depressive symptoms [109], and women with Borderline Personality Disorder [110].

6.5 Clinical Implication

Heightened awareness of the association between CSA and psychopathological outcomes, as well as of their etiological and maintaining factors, may improve health outcomes for abuse survivors. Survivors of sexual abuse use more medical care and incur greater costs than the general patient population [5]. A commonly shared observation is that CSA survivors represent a subpopulation of patients with specific maintaining factors of their symptoms, which are not efficaciously challenged by standard treatment interventions. Therefore these kinds of patients would show different response to treatment and long-term outcomes.

For example, depressive and anxiety disorders associated with a history of CSA have been found to respond differently to treatment [111] or are associated with treatment resistance [112]. In general, a history of child maltreatment is associated with significantly reduced efficacy for some **antidepressant medications** in depressed adults [97, 111]. A possible explanation is that patients with CSA are often comorbid with several different psychiatric conditions. Therefore, it is likely that a history of CSA reduces the efficacy of current treatments for other conditions such as substance abuse and impulse control disorders. Moreover, psychotherapy alone was found to be superior to antidepressant monotherapy [111].

Also standard psychotherapies are likely to be ineffective when CSA is part of the pathogenesis of a disorder. In a recent study, Castellini et al. [113] found that after a standard Cognitive Behavioral Therapy both Anorexia Nervosa and Bulimia Nervosa patients showed a significant improvement in terms of eating disorder psychopathology, as well as sexual functioning. However those patients reporting CSA did not show any improvement in body image disturbance and sexuality, showing a profound and different uneasiness in the relationship with one's own body as compared to other patients. Sanci et al. [8] proposed to always consider the possibility of sexual abuse when treatment of eating disorder does not follow the expected course or improvement. In general when the clinician assesses a history of CSA, he/she should specifically target the psychological consequences of the abuse before standard treatment can begin.

Psychotherapy may be an essential element in the treatment of patients with a history of CSA, and interventions that focus on childhood trauma may contribute to the development of more effective treatments for subgroups of disorders, preceded by childhood trauma. For example, in the case of eating disorders with CSA it is reasonable to hypothesize that a psychotherapy specifically targeted on body image perception and cognitive/emotional consequences of sexual abuse would improve the long-term outcome. Both group therapy and individual psychotherapy have been shown to improve psychological symptoms among sexual abuse survivors [114], and Habigzang et al. [115] demonstrated the efficacy of cognitive behavioural therapy in reducing symptoms of depression, anxiety, and PTSD in sexually abused girls.

References

1. Finkelhor D, Hotaling GT, Lewis IA, Smith C (1989) Sexual abuse and its relationship to later sexual satisfaction, marital status, religion, and attitudes. J Interpers Violence 4:379–399
2. Dunn EC, Gilman SE, Slopen N, Willett JB, Molnar BE (2012) The impact of exposure to interpersonal violence on gender differences in adolescent-onset major depression: results from the National Comorbidity Survey Replication (NCS-R). Depress Anxiety 29:392–399
3. Smolak L, Murnen SK (2002) A meta-analytic examination of the relationship between child sexual abuse and eating disorders. Int J Eat Disord 31:136–150
4. Maniglio R (2009) The impact of child sexual abuse on health: a systematic review of reviews. Clin Psychol Rev 29:647–657
5. Chen LP, Murad MH, Paras ML, Colbenson KM, Sattler AL, Goranson EN, Elamin MB, Seime RJ, Shinozaki G, Prokop LJ, Zirakzadeh A (2010) Sexual abuse and lifetime diagnosis of psychiatric disorders: systematic review and meta-analysis. Mayo Clin Proc 85:618–629
6. Carr CP, Martins CM, Stingel AM, Lemgruber VB, Juruena MF (2013) The role of early life stress in adult psychiatric disorders: a systematic review according to childhood trauma subtypes. J Nerv Ment Dis 201:1007–1020
7. Wonderlich SA, Brewerton TD, Jocic Z, Danskey BS, Abbott DW (1997) Relationship of childhood sexual abuse and eating disorders. J Am Acad Child Adolesc Psychiatry 36:1107–1115
8. Sanci L, Coffey C, Olsson C, Reid S, Carlin JB, Patton G (2008) Childhood sexual abuse and eating disorders in females: findings from the Victorian Adolescent Health Cohort Study. Arch Pediatr Adolesc Med 162:261–267

9. Zlotnick C, Johnson J, Kohn R, Vincente B, Rioseco P, Saldivia S (2008) Childhood trauma, trauma in adulthood, and psychiatric diagnoses: results from a community sample. Compr Psychiatry 49:163–169
10. Copeland WE, Keeler G, Angold A, Costello EJ (2007) Traumatic events and posttraumatic stress in childhood. Arch Gen Psychiatry 64:577–584
11. Faravelli C, Gorini Amedei S, Rotella F, Faravelli L, Palla A, Consoli G, Ricca V, Batini S, Lo Sauro C, Spiti A, Catena Dell'osso M (2010) Childhood traumata, Dexamethasone Suppression Test and psychiatric symptoms: a trans-diagnostic approach. Psychol Med 40:2037–2048
12. Mueller-Pfeiffer C, Moergeli H, Schumacher S, Martin-Soelch C, Wirtz G, Fuhrhans C, Hindermann E, Rufer M (2013) Characteristics of child maltreatment and their relation to dissociation, posttraumatic stress symptoms, and depression in adult psychiatric patients. J Nerv Ment Dis 201:471–477
13. Cutajar MC, Mullen PE, Ogloff JR, Thomas SD, Wells DL, Spataro J (2010) Psychopathology in a large cohort of sexually abused children followed up to 43 years. Child Abuse Negl 34:813–822
14. Jonas S, Bebbington P, McManus S, Meltzer H, Jenkins R, Kuipers E, Cooper C, King M, Brugha T (2011) Sexual abuse and psychiatric disorder in England: results from the 2007 Adult Psychiatric Morbidity Survey. Psychol Med 41:709–719
15. Wager-Smith K, Markou A (2011) Depression: a repair response to stress-induced neuronal microdamage that can grade into a chronic neuroinflammatory condition? Neurosci Biobehav Rev 35:742–764
16. Kessler RC, Chiu WT, Demler O, Merikangas KR, Walters EE (2005) Prevalence, severity, and comorbidity of 12-month DSM-IV disorders in the National Comorbidity Survey Replication. Arch Gen Psychiatry 62:617–627
17. Cicchetti D, Toth SL, Maughan A (2000) An ecological–transactional model of child maltreatment. In: Sameroff AJ, Lewis M, Miller SM (eds) Handbook of developmental psychopathology, 2nd edn. Kluwer/Plenum, New York, pp 689–722
18. Gibb BE, Chelminski I, Zimmerman M (2007) Childhood emotional, physical, and sexual abuse, and diagnoses of depressive and anxiety disorders in adult psychiatric outpatients. Depress Anxiety 24(4):256–263
19. Edwards VJ, Holden GW, Felitti VJ, Anda RF (2003) Relationship between multiple forms of childhood maltreatment and adult mental health in community respondents: results from the Adverse Childhood Experiences Study. Am J Psychiatry 160:1453–1460
20. Johnson J, Cohen P, Brown J, Smailes E, Bernstein D (1999) Childhood maltreatment increases risk for personality disorders during early adulthood. Arch Gen Psychiatry 56:600–609
21. van der Kolk B, Hostetler A, Herron N, Fisler R (1994) Trauma and the development of borderline personality disorder. Psychiatr Clin North Am 17:715–730
22. Westen D, Ludolph P, Misle B (1990) Physical and sexual abuse in adolescent girls with borderline personality disorder. Am J Orthopsychiatry 60:55–66
23. Horesh N, Nachshoni T, Wolmer L, Toren P (2009) A comparison of life events in suicidal and nonsuicidal adolescents and young adults with major depression and borderline personality disorder. Compr Psychiatry 50:496–502
24. Zanarini MC, Gunderson JG, Marino MF, Schwarz EO, Frankenburg FR (1989) Childhoood experience of borderline patients. Compr Psychiatry 30:18–25
25. Brown GW, Harris TO, Hepworth C (1994) Life events and endogenous depression. A puzzle reexamined. Arch Gen Psychiatry 51:525–534
26. Hovens JG, Wiersma JE, Giltay EJ, van Oppen P, Spinhoven P, Penninx BW, Zitman FG (2010) Childhood life events and childhood trauma in adult patients with depressive, anxiety and comorbid disorders vs. controls. Acta Psychiatr Scand 122:66–74
27. Fergusson D, Boden J, Horwood L (2008) Exposure to childhood sexual and physical abuse and adjustment in early adulthood. Child Abuse Negl 32:607–619

28. Gilbert R, Widom C, Browne K, Fergusson D, Webb E, Janson S (2009) Burden and consequences of child maltreatment in high-income countries. Lancet 373:68–81
29. Fergusson D, Horwood L, Lynskey M (1996) Childhood sexual abuse and psychiatric disorder in young adulthood. II. Psychiatric outcomes of childhood sexual abuse. J Am Acad Child Adolesc Psychiatry 34:1365–1374
30. Dinwiddie S, Heath AC, Dunne MP, Bucholz KK, Madden PA, Slutske WS, Bierut LJ, Statham DB, Martin NG (2000) Early sexual abuse and lifetime psychopathology: a co-twin study. Psychol Med 30:41–52
31. Klein DN, Shankman SA, Rose S (2006) Ten-year prospective follow-up study of the naturalistic course of dysthymic disorder and double depression. Am J Psychiatry 163:872–880
32. Fergusson D, Mullen P (1999) Childhood sexual abuse. An evidence based perspective. Sage, Thousand Oaks, CA
33. Andrews G, Corry J, Slade T, Issakidis C, Swanston H (2004) Child sexual abuse. Comparative quantification of health risks. WHO, Geneva
34. Kendall-Tackett K, Williams L, Finkelhor D (1993) Impact of sexual abuse on children: a review and synthesis of recent empirical studies. Psychol Bull 113:164–180
35. Rothman EF, Edwards EM, Heeren T, Hingson RW (2008) Adverse childhood experiences predict earlier age of drinking onset: results from a representative US sample of current or former drinkers. Pediatrics 122:e298–e304
36. Dube S, Anda R, Whitefield C, Brown D, Felitti V, Dong M, Giles WH (2005) Long-term consequences of childhood sexual abuse by gender of victim. Am J Prev Med 28:430–438
37. Bedi S, Nelson EC, Lynskey MT, McCutcheon VV, Heath AC, Madden PA, Martin NG (2011) Risk for suicidal thoughts and behavior after childhood sexual abuse in women and men. Suicide Life Threat Behav 41:406–415
38. Basile KC, Black MC, Simon TR, Arias R, Brener ND, Saltzman LE (2006) The association between selfreported lifetime history of forced sexual intercourse and recent health-risk behaviors: findings from the 2003 National Youth Risk Behavior Survey. J Adolesc Health 39:752.e1–752.e7
39. Hardt J, Sidor A, Nickel R, Kappis B, Petrak P, Egle UT (2008) Childhood adversities and suicide attempts: a retrospective study. J Fam Violence 23:713–718
40. Ullman SE, Najdowski CJ (2009) Correlates of serious suicidal ideation and attempts in female adult sexual assault survivors. Suicide Life Threat Behav 39:47–57
41. Peters DK, Range LM (1995) Childhood sexual abuse and current suicidality in college women and men. Child Abuse Negl 19:335–341
42. Jacobi C, Hayward C, de Zwaan M, Kraemer HC, Agras WS (2004) Coming to terms with risk factors for eating disorders: application of risk terminology and suggestions for a general taxonomy. Psychol Bull 130:19–65
43. Thompson KM, Wonderlich SA (2004) Child sexual abuse and eating disorders. In: Thompson KM (ed) Handbook of eating disorders and obesity. Wiley, Hoboken, NJ, pp 679–694
44. Johnson JG, Cohen P, Kasen S, Brook JS (2002) Childhood adversities associated with risk for eating disorders or weight problems during adolescence or early adulthood. Am J Psychiatry 159:394–400
45. Vanderlinden J, Van Dyck R, Vandereycken W, Vertommen H (1993) Dissociation and traumatic experiences in the general population of the Netherlands. Hosp Community Psychiatry 44:786–788
46. American Psychiatric Association (2002) Diagnostic and statistical manual of mental disorders, 4th edn., text rev. APA, Washington, DC
47. McManus F, Waller G (1995) A functional analysis of binge-eating. Clin Psychol Rev 15:845–863
48. Heatherton TF, Baumeister RF (1991) Binge eating as escape from selfawareness. Psychol Bull 110:86–108

49. Walker EA, Katon WJ, Neraas K, Jemelka RP, Massoth D (1992) Dissociation in women with chronic pelvic pain. Am J Psychiatry 149:534–537
50. Van der Hart O, Nijenhuis ER, Steele K, Brown D (2004) Trauma-related dissociation: conceptual clarity lost and found. Aust N Z J Psychiatry 38:906–914
51. Van der Kolk BA (2005) Developmental trauma disorder: toward a rational diagnosis for children with complex trauma histories. Psychiatr Ann 35:401–408
52. Chu JA, Frey LM, Ganzel BL, Matthews JA (1999) Memories of childhood abuse: dissociation, amnesia, and corroboration. Am J Psychiatry 156:749–755
53. Baron RM, Kenny DA (1986) The moderator-mediator variable distinction in social psychological research: conceptual, strategic, and statistical considerations. J Pers Soc Psychol 51(6):1173–1182
54. English DJ, Graham JC, Litrownik AJ, Everson M, Bangdiwala SI (2005) Defining maltreatment chronicity: are there differences in child outcomes. Child Abuse Negl 29:575–595
55. Dunn EC, McLaughlin KA, Slopen N, Rosand J, Smoller JW (2013) Developmental timing of child maltreatment and symptoms of depression and suicidal ideation in young adulthood: results from the National Longitudinal Study of Adolescent Health. Depress Anxiety 30:955–964
56. McCrory E, DeBrito SA, Viding E (2010) Research review: the neurobiology and genetics of maltreatment and adversity. J Child Psychol Psychiatry 51(10):1079–1095
57. McLaughlin KA, Greif Green J, Gruber MJ, Sampson NA, Zaslavsky AM, Kessler RC (2010) Childhood adversities and adult psychiatric disorders in the National Comorbidity Survey Replication II: associations with persistence of DSM-IV disorders. Arch Gen Psychiatry 67:124–132
58. Garbarino J (1989) Troubled youth, troubled families: the dynamics of adolescent maltreatment. In: Cicchetti D, Carlson V (eds) Child maltreatment: theory and research on the causes and consequences of child abuse and neglect. Cambridge University Press, NewYork, NY, pp 685–706
59. Cicchetti D (1989) How research on child maltreatment has informed the study of child development. In: Cicchetti D, Carlson V (eds) Child maltreatment: theory and research on the causes and consequences of child abuse and neglect. Cambridge University Press, New York, NY, pp 377–431
60. Kaplow J, Dodge K, Amaya-Jackson L, Saxe G (2005) Pathways to PTSD. Part II. Sexually abused children. Am J Psychiatry 162:1305–1310
61. Ehnvall A, Parker G, Hadzi-Pavlovic D, Malhi G (2008) Perception of rejecting and neglectful parenting in childhood relates to lifetime suicide attempts for females – but not for males. Acta Psychiatr Scand 117:50–56
62. Copeland WE, Magnusson A, Goransson M, Heilig MA (2011) Genetic moderators and psychiatric mediators of the link between sexual abuse and alcohol dependence. Drug Alcohol Depend 115:183–189
63. Schultz T, Passmore JL, Yoder CY (2003) Emotional closeness with perpetrators and amnesia for child sexual abuse. J Child Sex Abus 12:67–88
64. Van der Hart O, Nijenhuis ER, Steele K (2006) The haunted self. Structural dissociation and the treatment of chronic traumatization. W W Norton, New York, NY
65. Heller SS, Larrieu JA, D'Imperio R, Boris NW (1999) Research on resilience to child maltreatment: empirical considerations. Child Abuse Negl 23:321–338
66. Sperry DM, Widom CS (2013) Child abuse and neglect, social support, and psychopathology in adulthood: a prospective investigation. Child Abuse Negl 37:415–425
67. Cohen S, Gottlieb BH, Underwood LG (2000) Social relationships and health. In: Cohen S, Underwood LG, Gottlieb BH (eds) Social support measurement and intervention: a guide for health and social scientists. Oxford University Press, New York, NY, pp 3–25
68. Cohen S, Hoberman HM (1983) Positive events and social supports as buffers of life change stress. J Appl Soc Psychol 13:99–125

69. Feldman BJ, Conger RD, Burzette RG (2004) Traumatic events, psychiatric disorders, and pathways to risk and resilience during the transition to adulthood. Res Hum Dev 1:259–290
70. Hyman SM, Gold SN, Cott MA (2003) Forms of social support that moderate PTSD in childhood sexual abuse survivors. J Fam Violence 18:295–300
71. Kaniasty KZ, Norris FH (1993) A test of the social support deterioration model in the context of natural disaster. J Pers Soc Psychol 64:395–408
72. Widom CS, Czaja SJ, Dutton MA (2008) Childhood victimization and lifetime revictimization. Child Abuse Negl 32:785–796
73. Rosenman S, Rodgers B (2004) Childhood adversity in an Australian population. Soc Psychiatry Psychiatr Epidemiol 39:695–702
74. Anda RF, Felitti VJ, Bremner JD, Walker JD, Whitfield C, Perry BD, Dube SR, Giles WH (2006) The enduring effects of abuse and related adverse experiences in childhood. A convergence of evidence from neurobiology and epidemiology. Eur Arch Psychiatry Clin Neurosci 256:174–186
75. Favaro A, Tenconi E, Santonastaso P (2010) The interaction between perinatal factors and childhood abuse in the risk of developing anorexia nervosa. Psychol Med 40:657–665
76. Caspi A, Sugden K, Moffitt TE, Taylor A, Craig IW, Harrington H, McClay J, Mill J, Martin J, Braithwaite A, Poulton R (2003) Influence of life stress on depression: moderation by a polymorphism in the 5-HTT gene. Science 301:386–389
77. Kendler KS, Kuhn JW, Vittum J, Prescott CA, Riley B (2005) The interaction of stressful life events and a serotonin transporter polymorphism in the prediction of episodes of major depression: a replication. Arch Gen Psychiatry 62:529–535
78. Kaufman J, Yang BZ, Douglas-Palumberi H, Grasso D, Lipschitz D, Houshyar S, Krystal JH, Gelernter J (2006) Brain-derived neurotrophic factor-5-HTTLPR gene interactions and environmental modifiers of depression in children. Biol Psychiatry 59:673–680
79. Cicchetti D, Rogosch FA, Sturge-Apple ML (2007) Interactions of child maltreatment and serotonin transporter and monoamine oxidase A polymorphisms: depressive symptomatology among adolescents from low socioeconomic status backgrounds. Dev Psychopathol 19:1161–1180
80. Steiger H, Richardson J, Joober R, Gauvin L, Israel M, Bruce KR, Ying Kin NM, Howard H, Young SN (2007) The 5HTTLPR polymorphism, prior maltreatment, and dramatic-erratic personality manifestations in women with bulimic syndromes. J Psychiatry Neurosci 32:354–362
81. Steiger H, Richardson J, Joober R, Israel M, Bruce KR, Ng Ying Kin NM, Howard H, Anestin A, Dandurand C, Gauvin L (2008) Dissocial behavior, the 5HTTLPR polymorphism and maltreatment in women with bulimic syndromes. Am J Med Genet B 147B:128–130
82. Kumsta R, Entringer S, Koper JW, van Rossum EF, Hellhammer DH, Wüst S (2007) Sex specific associations between common glucocorticoid receptor gene variants and hypothalamus-pituitary-adrenal axis responses to psychosocial stress. Biol Psychiatry 62:863–869
83. Wüst S, Federenko IS, van Rossum EF, Koper JW, Kumsta R, Entringer S, Hellhammer DH (2004) A psychobiological perspective on genetic determinants of hypothalamuspituitary-adrenal axis activity. Ann NY Acad Sci 1032:52–62
84. Steiger H, Gauvin L, Joober R, Israel M, Badawi G, Groleau P, Bruce KR, Yin Kin NM, Sycz L, Ouelette AS (2012) Interaction of the BcII glucocorticoid receptor polymorphism and childhood abuse in bulimia nervosa (BN): relationship to BN and to associated trait manifestations. J Psychiatr Res 46:152–158
85. Bradley RG, Binder EB, Epstein MP, Tang Y, Nair HP, Liu W, Gillespie CF, Berg T, Evces M, Newport DJ, Stowe ZN, Heim CM, Nemeroff CB, Schwartz A, Cubells JF, Ressler KJ (2008) Influence of child abuse on adult depression: moderation by the corticotropin-releasing hormone receptor gene. Arch Gen Psychiatry 65:190–200
86. Binder EB, Bradley RG, Liu W, Epstein MP, Deveau TC, Mercer KB, Tang Y, Gillespie CF, Heim CM, Nemeroff CB, Schwartz AC, Cubells JF, Ressler KJ (2008) Association of FKBP5

polymorphisms and childhood abuse with risk of posttraumatic stress disorder symptoms in adults. JAMA 299:1291–1305
87. Gamble SA, Talbot NL, Duberstein PR, Conner KR, Franus N, Beckman AM, Conwell Y (2006) Childhood sexual abuse and depressive symptom severity: the role of neuroticism. J Nerv Ment Dis 194:382–385
88. Ormel J, Riese H, Rosmalen JG (2012) Interpreting neuroticism scores across the adult life course: immutable or experience-dependent set points of negative affect? Clin Psychol Rev 32:71–79
89. Martin G, Bergen HA, Richardson AS, Roeger L, Allison S (2004) Sexual abuse and suicidality: gender differences in a large community sample of adolescents. Child Abuse Negl 28:491–503
90. Sigfusdottir ID, Asgeirsdottir BB, Gudjonsson GH, Sigurdsson JF (2008) A model of sexual abuse's effects on suicidal behavior and delinquency: the role of emotions as mediating factors. J Youth Adolesc 37:699–712
91. Ferraz L, Vallez M, Navarro JB, Gelabert E, Martin-Santos R, Subirà S (2009) Dimensional assessment of personality and impulsiveness in borderline personality disorder. Pers Indiv Differ 46:140–146
92. Ladd C, Huot R, Thrivikraman K, Nemeroff C, Meaney M, Plotsky P (2000) Long-term behavioral and neuroendocrine adaptations to adverse early experience. Prog Brain Res 122:81–103
93. Burns EE, Fischer S, Jackson JL, Harding HG (2012) Deficits in emotion regulation mediate the relationship between childhood abuse and later eating disorder symptoms. Child Abuse Negl 36:32–39
94. Kraus ED, Mendelson T, Lynch TR (2003) Childhood emotional invalidation and adult psychological distress: the mediating role or emotional inhibition. Child Abuse Negl 27:199–213
95. Gratz KL, Bornovalova MA, Delany-Brumsey A, Nick B, Lejuez CW (2007) A laboratory-based study of the relationship between childhood abuse and experiential avoidance among inner-city substance users: the role of emotional nonacceptance. Behav Ther 38:256–268
96. Bowlby J (1969) Attachment and loss. Basic Books, New York, NY
97. Putnam KT, Harris WW, Putnam FW (2013) Synergistic childhood adversities and complex adult psychopathology. J Trauma Stress 26:435–442
98. Arnow B, Kennedy J, Agras WS (1992) Binge eating among the obese: a descriptive study. J Behav Med 15:155–170
99. Preti A, Incani E, Camboni MV, Petretto DR, Masala C, Lockwood R, Lawson R, Waller G (2004) Compulsive features in the eating disorders: a role for trauma? J Nerv Ment Dis 192:247–249
100. Kearney-Cooke A, Ackard DM (2000) The effects of sexual abuse on body image, self-image, and sexual activity of women. J Gend Specif Med 3:54–60
101. Ackard DM, Kearney-Cooke A, Peterson CB (2000) Effect of body image and self-image on women's sexual behaviors. Int J Eat Disord 28:422–429
102. Pujols Y, Cindy MM, Seal Brooke N (2010) The association between sexual satisfaction and body image in women. J Sex Med 7:905–916
103. La Rocque CI, Cioe J (2010) An evaluation of the relationship between body image and sexual avoidance. J Sex Res 47:1–12
104. Sanchez DT, Kiefer AK (2007) Body concerns in and out of the bedroom: implications for sexual pleasure and problems. Arch Sex Behav 36:808–820
105. Pinheiro AP, Raney TJ, Thornton LM, Fichter MM, Berrettini WH, Goldman D, Halmi KA, Kaplan AS, Strober M, Treasure J, Woodside DB, Kaye WH, Bulik CM (2010) Sexual functioning in women with eating disorders. Int J Eat Disord 43:123–129
106. Rellini AH, Meston CM (2009) The cortisol response during physiological sexual arousal in adult women with a history of childhood sexual abuse. J Trauma Stress 22:557–565

107. Bremner JD, Vythilingam M, Vermetten E, Adil J, Khan S, Nazeer A, Afzal N, McGlashan T, Elzinga B, Anderson GM, Heninger G, Southwick SM, Charney DS (2003) Cortisol response to a cognitive stress challenge in posttraumatic stress disorder (PTSD) related to childhood abuse. Psychoneuroendocrinology 28:733–750
108. Newport DJ, Heim C, Bonsall R, Miller AH, Nemeroff CB (2004) Pituitary–adrenal responses to standard and low dose dexamethasone suppression tests in adult survivors of child abuse. Biol Psychiatry 55:10–20
109. Heim C, Mletzko T, Purselle D, Musselman DL, Nemeroff CB (2008) The dexamethasone/corticotropin-releasing factor test in men with major depression: role of childhood trauma. Biol Psychiatry 63:398–405
110. Rinne T, de Kloet ER, Wouters L, Goekoop JG, DeRijk RH, van den Brink W (2008) Hyperresponsiveness of hypothalamic-pituitary-adrenal axis to combined mexamethasone/corticotropin-releasing hormone challenge in female borderline personality disorder subjects with a history of sustained childhood abuse. Biol Psychiatry 52:1102–1112
111. Nemeroff CB, Heim CM, Thase ME, Klein DN, Rush AJ, Schatzberg AF, Ninan PT, McCullough JP Jr, Weiss PM, Dunner DL, Rothbaum BO, Kornstein S, Keitner G, Keller MB (2003) Differential responses to psychotherapy versus pharmacotherapy in patients with chronic forms of major depression and childhood trauma. Proc Natl Acad Sci U S A 100:14293–14296
112. Kaplan MJ, Klinetob NA (2000) Childhood emotional trauma and chronic posttraumatic stress disorder in adult outpatients with treatment-resistant depression. J Nerv Ment Dis 188:596–601
113. Castellini G, Lo Sauro C, Lelli L, Godini L, Vignozzi L, Rellini AH, Faravelli C, Maggi M, Ricca V (2013) Childhood sexual abuse moderates the relationship between sexual functioning and eating disorder psychopathology in anorexia nervosa and bulimia nervosa: a 1-year follow-up study. J Sex Med 10:2190–2200
114. Ryan M, Nitsun M, Gilbert L, Mason H (2005) A prospective study of the effectiveness of group and individual psychotherapy for women CSA survivors. Psychol Psychother 78:465–479
115. Habigzang LF, Stroeher FH, Hatzenberger R, Cunha RC, Ramos Mda S, Koller SH (2009) Cognitive behavioral group therapy for sexually abused girls. Rev Saude Publica 43(Suppl 1):70–78

Atypical Sexual Offenders

7

Daniele Mollaioli, Erika Limoncin, Giacomo Ciocca, and Emmanuele A. Jannini

7.1 Female Paedophilia

7.1.1 Introduction

If talking about paedophilia evokes extremely strong and "disturbing" feelings, as any other type of male-related paraphilia does, the effect of discussing **female paedophilia** is even greater. Female paedophilia is mainly a sore spot, an uncomfortable phenomenon disrupting those rational, social, cultural and emotional certainties that make up the existence of each of us: motherhood and the physical and mental development of the child.

Imagining a "sexually active" woman in terms of both desires/fantasies and acted out behaviours has always been a sort of "taboo". Consequently, foreseeing female paedophilia complicates everything: it represents a sort of "**taboo of taboos**" just because women, in addition to violating the incest taboo, violate an even more serious taboo—the unfinished and disowned maternity.

Paedophilia in women is therefore such a rare clinical phenomenon that its existence has even been questioned by some researchers [1, 2], and even when studied, investigation has been based on discussions of clinical cases rather than on real large-scale research [3].

Indeed, female paedophilia seems always to have existed and is therefore not an innovation of modern times. Formerly (2,000 years ago), Petronius described in his

---

D. Mollaioli • E. Limoncin • G. Ciocca
Department of Biotecnological and Applied Clinical Sciences, University of L'Aquila, Via Vetoio, L'Aquila 67100, Italy
e-mail: daniele.mollaioli@gmail.com; erika.limoncin@gmail.com; giacomo.ciocca@libero.it

E.A. Jannini (✉)
Department of Systems Medicine, University of Rome Tor Vergata, Rome, Italy
e-mail: eajannini@gmail.com

Satyricon a group of women cheering in front of the rape of a 7-year-old girl. In the past there was a form of paedophilia or "paederasty" interpreted as entirely "feminine".

Furthermore, often the analysis of female paedophilia is extended to topics that do not fit so explicitly in the context, despite apparently being very connected. Analysis usually deals with criminal women, women and sex tourism, Munchausen syndrome, self-harm, anorexia and kleptomania. These clinical conditions share with female paedophilia the fact that a woman is involved in acts of "aggression" (Munchausen syndrome and women criminals). Those acts are typically sexually deviant behaviours associated with men (sex tourism with children and adolescents) that should not, according to a collective and stereotypical imaginary, belong to women.

Indeed, female paedophilia is another condition altogether; the risk lies in putting very different phenomena indiscriminately into a single cauldron.

7.1.2 Prevalence Data

Female paedophilia, as highlighted by the scientific literature, is a phenomenon apparently much less frequent than male paedophilia. This is certainly due to a lower frequency of the real phenomenon, but also to a "bio-psycho-social" discourse: in the Occident, women have always played a more "passive and soft" role compared to men, who are considered far more "active and hard".

This mindset involves the risk of not wanting to look at the contexts in which female paedophilia may be present. A significant portion of female paedophilia is therefore "**submerged**" because it is more difficult to detect, most often masked and certainly less studied than male paedophilia.

In the 2008 report of the U.S. National Center for Missing and Exploited Children, in a sample of 731,584 abused children, 65 % had suffered attitudes of negligence from their parents, 10 % had suffered physical abuse (beatings and negligence) and 2.3 % had suffered sexual abuse. 58 % of offenders were female, with two peaks in the 20–29 age range (41.3 %) and the 30–39 age range (36.7 %), compared with 42.1 % of the offenders being men (age range 20–29: 28.9 %, 30–39: 36.2 % and 40–49: 21.3 %).

In other researches about female paedophilia, researchers reveal an even higher percentage. As reported by Welldon [4], in 1994 the National Opinion Research Center showed that the second most common form of child sexual abuse was committed by women who molest boys. Specifically, for every three instances of abuse by men, there is one by a woman. This data was recently confirmed by Childline [5] (a childcare-based organisation that also runs a friend line for troubled children) which, on the basis of requests for assistance received by children in 2008 (2,142 requests), asserts that child sexual abuse by women represents **25 % of all the cases** with which it deals.

Online paedophilia is also rising. At the beginning of 2004, there were only five associations for paedophilic women on the Internet, but by 2007 this number had increased to 36, as reported by the Meter, an agency which has been dealing with the phenomenon of paedophilia for several years [6].

7.1.3 Characteristics of Female Paedophilia

The woman, as a mother, spends most of the day especially in the first phase of the development of her child [7], focusing particularly on "physical" cares. In this extremely intimate and ambiguous context of care—at an erotic and sexual level—female paedophilia can be expressed by many "**disguises**". According to Welldon [4], female perversions realised through motherhood and the pervasive use of manipulative strategies on the child, rather than through sexuality.

The mother can, in fact, engage in sexual acts with her child through frequent and prolonged baby baths, for example, in which the mother's hands hesitate longer than necessary on the child's genitals, or while sleeping together in bed or taking a bath together naked by taking advantage of that "healthy" contextual situation to be touched in intimate areas usually procuring sexual arousal.

Such activities definitely involve an extreme abuse of power, because a mother has total control over her son, even more than a father has.

According to Petrone [8–10], female paedophiles can be divided into "types" on the basis of their **personality characteristics**:

- *Latent*: those who have a strong sex drive toward children, but because of social and legal restrictions do not manifest that drive in any overt behaviour.
- *Occasional*: for these paedophiles the paedophilic behaviour occurs only when external conditions can facilitate it: for example, when the paedophile is in foreign countries that hinder or condemn paedophilia less than her home country does.
- *Immature*: among such individuals there is basically a lack of development of an adult psychosexuality and age-appropriate interpersonal skills.
- *Regressive*: these individuals have reached a normal adult psychosexual development, but in high emotional stress situations can manifest behaviours associated with paedophiles.
- *Aggressive*: individuals with low self-esteem and a strong sense of powerlessness that can lead to real "sadism" against the victim.

There is also a particular form of paedophilic expression that Petrone [9, 10] defines as "**pre-paedophilia**". This term indicates the shrewd, complex and perverse dynamic that arises when the woman/mother does not directly engage in paedophilic behaviours towards her child, but becomes the "accomplice" of those who really abuse the child (usually the mother's partners). This is a phenomenon that could be called "**compulsion to see repeated**": it is like the Freudian mechanism of the repetition compulsion, only filtered by the active presence of another person who does the dirty work for someone else. Ignoring the abuse is a further act of violence against young unprotected and abused victims by those who should love and protect them.

Betrayal happens on all fronts and the child is left alone. These women, despite not having committed a direct abuse, are guilty of the same crime as their partners because, just like those partners, they have not considered the children as human beings, have frustrated and maimed their physical and mental development and bent them to their unjustified and irrational demands.

Pre-paedophilia has different manifestations: it can be shrewd, silent and masked, as in **incestuous families**, or be more obvious, more ostentatious, as in the case of mothers who "push" their children towards their fellow abusers, or "sell" performances of their children or are actively involved in perverse sexual games with them.

Following the classification of Petrone [9, 10], there are at least three **types of pre-paedophilic** women/mothers:

- The *collusive mother* is the ultimate expression of the pre-paedophilic female. This kind of mother, unconsciously but also consciously, sacrifices her child to a full-blown paedophile, thus satisfying her need to attack and humiliate the child while remaining in a passive position.
- The *dependent mother* has an extremely fragile personality. She is therefore not able to perform her biological role of protector of her children and has no power within the family, but is totally subordinate to her partner.
- The *victim mother* is stuck in the abuser–abused cycle, so this kind of women, as demonstrated by many studies in the past, was herself a victim of sexual abuse. In this case, in addition to the unconscious motivation to harm someone else in ways similar to what she suffered in childhood, the woman puts in place the well-known **defence mechanisms** of denial, repression and displacement, so the devastating emotions related to incest by another family member are not recognised and therefore somehow removed.

In this regard, pre-paedophilia is actually the only significant difference between female and male paedophilia. Pre-paedophilia seems to be a characteristic of women only.

In addition, according to Welldon [4], the woman has as her primary objective damaging herself through the other, which is different from the motivation of the man, who actively retaliates against others in response to a personal experience of abuse in childhood. The act of abusing children, then, has for a woman the same meaning as abusing against herself. Especially in cases of abusive women who have previously been abused, they inevitably internalise their own hated mothers in their female bodies and identify with their children's bodies. The female paedophile tends to see herself as an extension of her own child, much as she has been treated in the past as an extension of her mother. So we can talk about female paedophilia in terms of "**self-directed**" aggression.

7.1.4 Conclusions

In conclusion, the explanation for female paedophilia when there are no severe psychiatric dysfunctions can be traced back to the "**abuser–abused cycle**" [11]. In this case, the women unleashed their anger, accumulated in the past because of abuses they suffered, through many kinds of offending behaviours directed towards their children.

Abusive women, like abusive men, compromise profound aspects of their existence, but they also specifically compromise their maternal role, allowing themselves to violate their children by enabling forms of incest, but mostly behaviour that is detrimental to the emotional, cognitive and psychological development of their children [12, 13].

As well as the discussion presented here suggests, the greatest **issue** recognised by the scientific community related to the understanding not only of the characteristics associated with feminine paedophilia, but especially the prevalence and the escalation of the phenomenon related to the inability to study significant samples of women paedophiles. This is not just because there is a lower prevalence of female paedophilia than there is of male paedophilia, but mostly because women paedophiles belong to a **hidden phenomenon** and full of disguises.

7.2 Sexual Offenders with Intellectual Disabilities: From the Role of Victim to the Role of Aggressor

7.2.1 Introduction

The sexuality of people affected by intellectual disabilities has for long been considered a troublesome argument. The difficulty involved in addressing this topic is probably due to the perception of a person affected by intellectual disabilities as an asexual individual, or as an individual with the potential to be sexually dangerous. *Vice versa*, it was also discovered the existence of a group of individuals sexually attracted by physical and/or intellectual disabilities [14]. These individuals define themselves as "*devotees*" [14].

Nowadays it is possible to note the historical importance that intellectual disability has held and the **prejudice** with which it has been understood in views on crime and the criminal justice service [15, 16]. Many people with **intellectual disabilities (ID)** may express their sexual needs in an inappropriate manner: for example, they might live their sexuality in a social context, rather than a private one. The expression of this problematic behaviour is probably caused by the absence of specific sexual education programmes that take account of intellectually disabled people's cognitive difficulties. The opportunity to learn appropriate modalities to satisfy their own sexual needs might prevent the imprisonment of people with ID for moral deficiencies. In this manner, the problem of the increasing prevalence of offenders with ID in prisons or mental hospitals, who moreover are institutionalised for indefinite periods, could be resolved.

7.2.2 Prevalence Rates and Characteristics of Sex Offenders with Intellectual Disabilities

Prevalence rates of legal involvement regarding people affected by ID are uncertain data, because of their variation across the literature [17]. This variability is probably due to significant methodological differences between studies [16]. In particular, difficulties might arise with the definition of ID and legal criteria. Moreover, it should be considered that some intellectually disabled people's caregivers could hesitate in reporting criminal offences [18]. However, scientific evidence generally highlights that 5–15 % of persons with ID come into conflict with the **law** [17]. This frequency appears to be less than 5–15 % only in one study conducted in prisons in Victoria, Australia [19].

Regarding characteristics configuring the **average sex offender** with ID, evidence shows differences between **forensic and non-forensic samples** [20]. Sex offenders with ID belonging to the forensic group seem to be younger and predominantly male. They often report histories of **substance abuse** and **psychiatric comorbidities**, with the exception of mood disorder. With respect to cognitive level, data show the prevalence of mild intellectual disabilities or borderline intelligence among forensic sex offenders.

Many studies have shown the presence of some variables concurring in the expression of sexually deviant behaviour among people affected by ID. What often emerges is the association of sexually deviant behaviour with high rates of childhood neglect, physical health problems, adult mental health problems and perinatal adversities [21]. In addition, other studies found the prevalence of attention deficit hyperactivity disorder (ADHD) in sexual offenders with ID [22]. Discordant opinions remain with respect to the theory of the sexual offender who has also been sexually abused. The first studies investigating the presence of sexual abuse among adult sex offenders found prevalence rates between 18 and 58 % [23–25]. However, these preliminary data have not been confirmed by other research [26, 27]. In particular, it was shown that the number of sex offences committed by individuals who have been sexually abused in childhood is interchangeable with that of sex offenders who have never been sexually abused [27]. In addition, no differences were found between sex offenders and non-sex offenders regarding the presence of physical abuse in childhood. Hence, the hypothesis that sexual abuse in childhood is the primary pathway to sexual offending in adulthood is probably a reductive thought. However, it is possible to suppose that people who have experienced different kinds of abuse in childhood—physical or sexual—may manifest their negative emotional experiences by utilising the coping strategy of sexual or non-sexual offences [28].

7.2.3 The Hypothesised Existence of Two Types of Sex Offenders with Intellectual Disabilities

An understanding of the significance of sexual offending is necessary to a consideration of the diagnostic criteria of sexual deviance, better known as paraphilia. The Diagnostic and Statistical Manual of Mental Disorders (**DSM-5, pp 685**) defines **paraphilia** as "any intense and persistent sexual interest other than sexual interest in genital stimulation or preparatory fondling with phenotypically normal, physically mature, consenting human partners" [29]. However, the definition of paraphilia is not applicable to all cases of sexual offending on the part of persons affected by ID. For this reason, some authors have proposed the existence of two subpopulations of sex offenders with ID: one subpopulation characterised by offenders who are similar to mainstream offenders and who appear to fit the label of paraphilia, and the second subpopulation of offenders composed of individuals who are sexually inappropriate in their behaviour but have the tendency to commit minor or nuisance offences [30]. In addition, it was hypothesised that the principal motivation for committing sexual offences among the second subset of individuals are not the recurring urges or fantasies that typify paraphilia. On the contrary, sexual offending caused by a "**counterfeit deviance**" seems prevalent among such individuals. With this term some authors have proposed the existence of a deviant sexual behaviour which is not associated with sexual fantasies or urges, or the intention either to harm or humiliate others [31]. On the contrary, counterfeit deviance might emerge as a consequence of the life experiences of some persons with ID, such as socio-environmental or social learning conditions, a lack of communication skills, or a lack of socio-sexual knowledge regarding privacy/boundaries [32]. This hypothesis permits the consideration of sexual offending as a result of a lack of normative learning experiences, and the presence of segregation, imposed restrictions or social attitudes tending to infantilise individuals with ID, rather than as a result of deviant sexual urges. At the same time, as shown by Michie et al. [33] and Talbot and Langdon [34], persons with ID whose sexual offending fulfils the criteria of paraphilia have in most cases more advanced sexual knowledge than other individuals with ID. This knowledge is probably attributable to previous sex education courses in which sex offenders with ID had to participate due to a penal sanction.

A lack of sexual knowledge or, in a more general view, socio-environmental conditions may play a role in some kinds of sexual offences. Hence, only a scrupulous differential diagnosis might reveal if sexual offending is caused by deviant sexual urges and fantasies, or by other factors.

7.2.4 Assessment

The assessment of variables implicated in the development of sexual offending is an argument well investigated in many previous studies. The work on risk assessment for sex offenders with ID is different. In fact, some authors [35] have questioned the validity of existing risk assessment scales and methods for the quantification of the risk of sexual offending in people with ID.

As suggested by Camilleri and Quinsey [36], the central point is not only the investigation and the identification of risk factors implied in the development of sexual offending among individuals with ID, but also the establishment of their effectiveness as predictors of the risk of reoffending.

Regarding the global evaluation of the incidence of sexual offending on the part of individuals with ID, the evidence found in the literature suggests the adoption of the Violence Risk Appraisal Guide (**VRAG**) [37].

However, the assessment of sex offenders with ID cannot exclude the evaluation of other variables concurring in defining the extent of the sexual deviance. One of the most important variables considered in the assessment of sex offenders with ID is personality disorder. Generally, this variable seems to have predictive validity and structural validity with individuals with ID. The association between VRAG scores and the presence of Antisocial Personality Disorder was also shown, as was the association between Antisocial Personality Disorder and other risk assessments [37]. Another factor bearing on the development of sexual offending is the presence of externalising emotional problems.

In some cases it was supposed that the absence of adequate sexual knowledge might lead to the deviant externalisation of sexual needs. The instrument proposed to explore this variable is the Socio-Sexual Knowledge and Attitudes Assessment Tool—Revised (**SSKAAT-R**) [38]. This tool permits a comprehensive assessment of areas of socio-sexual knowledge and attitudes among people with ID. However, poor sexual knowledge, as a single factor, might not cause sexual offending on the part of individuals with ID. Instead, this lack might act only as a contributing factor.

Literature shows that an intellectually disabled forensic population does not have a secure attachment to primary caregivers and presents a high prevalence of low self-esteem [39]. For this reason, it may be advantageous to evaluate self-esteem in this group. The instrument used for detecting self-esteem in a population of subjects affected by ID is the six-item version of the **Rosenberg Self-Esteem Scale** [39]. This tool aims to measure feelings of self-acceptance, self-respect and positive self-evaluation.

Other hypotheses were developed to explain why some individuals with ID commit sexual offences. A factor determining the inability to understand the negative effect produced by their deviant behaviour is a deficit in empathy. Although the correlation of an empathy deficit with sexual offending remains contradictory [40], treatments of sex offenders provide empathy training in most cases.

Finally, the assessment of sex offenders with ID should comprehend the evaluation of the **risk of reoffending**. In fact, by verifying the presence of some specific variables, it is possible to predict which sex offenders with ID are at a major risk of reoffending. These variables are previous drug offences, previous bail offences, the number of previous offences, a history of alcohol abuse, previous acquisitive offences, an antisocial attitude, a lack of assertiveness, low self-esteem, a poor relationship with the mother, allowances made by staff, staff complacency, and a poor response to treatment. A suggested tool for the evaluation of the risk of reoffending is the **Offender Group Reconviction Scale** [37].

7.2.5 Treatment Essentials

Scientific literature on the treatment of sex offenders with ID is still scarce. The first treatment methods for these individuals adopted a pharmacological approach. In fact, there were suggestions about the efficacy of antiandrogen cyproterone (**CPA**) or antiandrogen medroxyprogesterone (**MPA**) in decreasing the intensity and frequency of sexual fantasies and sexual behaviours [41]. However, neither of these drugs has been approved by the Food and Drug Administration in the United States.

Other treatment hypotheses were suggested in the past for the prevention of reoffending behaviours. Among these are included psycho-social interventions (skills training and behavioural therapy) as well as less permitted treatments (covert sensitisation, olfactory aversion and electrical aversion therapy) [42].

Nowadays, the treatment receiving a significant scientific consensus is the cognitive-behavioural treatment (**CBT**), the aim of which is to reduce a client's sexually abusive behaviour [43]. The procedure comprises: (1) a social therapeutic framework (establishing group rules, addressing initial denial and developing group social skills); (2) human relations and sex education (understanding sexuality and relationships, and understanding consent and legal issues); (3) the cognitive model (changing the client's cognitive distortions which cause the sexually abusive behaviour); (4) victim empathy (development of empathy to regulate and mediate pro-social behaviour); and (5) relapse prevention (preventing recidivism or failure of maintenance).

Recently it has been proposed the application of mindfulness procedures to treat and prevent sexual offending [44]. In particular, **mindfulness-based procedures** were utilised to reduce deviant sexual arousal in three case studies, disengaging the clients from their sexual thoughts. The surprising result of this study evidenced the significant reduction of self-rated arousal after 60 weeks.

7.2.6 Conclusions

Although little is still known about sexual offending perpetrated by individuals with ID, some research highlights the utility of better comprehending this phenomenon. The key points in need of in-depth analysis are the assessment of dynamic risk for offenders with ID and the evaluation of treatment effects in broader populations. In this manner, research might contribute to both a reduction in offending/reoffending and the implementation of a socio-sexual quality of life for sex offenders with ID.

7.3 Sexual Abuse in the Context of Religion and Spirituality

7.3.1 Introduction

The vast majority of acts of violence and abuse pertain to a paradoxical dimension: the abuser is often a person who should play a leading role or even a caregiver. Sexual abuses are often perpetrated by family members such as fathers, mothers, grandfathers or uncles who commit an intolerable crime against the designated victim [45].

Sexual abuse and violence also occur in other situational contexts, where it is not parenting that is associated with abusive acting out but a spiritual bond.

Myth, religion and spiritual contexts are crowded with scenes, stories, tales and dramatic reported cases of acts of sexual violence [46].

Western history has never concealed this macabre aspect of myth, as if to prove that spiritual practices are also strongly dominated by aspects of perversity.

Greek myth, through the cult of **Dionysus**, transmitted to the Western Culture a combination of divinity, violence and sexuality in which a sacrificial victim is always present [47, 48]. Also, Jewish-Christian tradition reports cruel events characterised by fratricide, brutality and divine sacrifices. The biblical characters of Cain and Abel and Abraham and Isaac are clear examples. In this chapter, it will be analysed the phenomenon of abuse in the main religious context: in Judaism, in Christian churches, in Muslim religion, in Hinduism, and in satanism.

7.3.2 Christian Churches

Two psychologists, **Mary Frawley-O'Dea** and **Virginia Goldner**, have carefully studied the issue of sexual abuse by catholic clergy, collecting prominent contributions and analysing literature and studies on this topic [49].

The main point of reference of the two researchers was the *John Jay Study*. This report determined that over 4 % of American priests have committed sexual abuse and that from 1950 to about 2004, nearly 11,000 individuals have been sexually abused by clergy [49]. Actually, many believe that these figures are much lower than the real ones and that most instances of abuse are being covered up and hushed up to avoid scandal and protect the reputation of the Catholic Church.

Denial is deemed to be the main defence mechanism adopted by the Church to protect itself from all abuse charges levied against abusive priests.

Whereas data resulting from the *John Jay Study* pertain to the American Church, with the ***Murphy Report***, released in 2009, the scourge of sexual abuse arrived in Europe, disconcerting the Irish Church. One year later, Germany was involved in a similar scandal.

Frawley-O'Dea and Goldner clarify that child sexual abuse by priests is favoured by power relations, by an essential misogyny and by a narcissist's sense of omnipotence that may be typical of the priestly personality. The criminal act can also be induced by a sexually repressive education and the pathological psychosexual immaturity of the sex offender. Moreover, sexual orientation does not influence the criminal behaviour of a paedophile and having been abused during childhood does not seem to be a predictive factor of sexual offending among catholic priests.

Nevertheless, Catholicism does not represent the only Christian community affected from these terrible histories. Also the Orthodox, Protestant and Anglican churches were been crossed by cases of youth people abused. An Australian Web site showed the misconducts of 18 Anglican ministers who were been authors of sexual abuse on child [50]. In this survey, the authors hypothesised a major prevalence of sexual abuse in women than men, due substantially to the possibility of marriage for priest. Instead, also in Anglican Church the most of abuses were perpetrated in youth males. The author of this investigation concludes that is suitable collaboration among Anglican, other Protestant and Catholic churches to prevent the abuses on child [50].

7.3.3 Judaism

Judaism is the first monotheistic religion characterised by some obsessions and several prohibitions related to reproduction, sexuality and marriage. Are these characteristics directly or indirectly cause of neurotic and perverse symptoms, as literarily suggested in the *Portnoy's Complaint* [51]. It could be even hypothesised that hardly psychoanalysis would arbour outside the repressive and matriarchal background of Judaism. The Freud's Hebraic origins is far to be casual in the genesis of the psychodynamic theories [52].

In the Hebraic culture, the gender roles are clearly defined. In the **Torah**, sexual relations between people of the same sex are forbidden, demonstrating a clear tendency towards discrimination. The female gender is also discriminated against, with women being forbidden from frequenting the Synagogue [53]. In this regard, Judaism could be considered a multi-form religion, composed of many positions regarding gender roles in society and in the religious life. Are the above-mentioned forms of discrimination against women and homosexuals to be considered forms of psychological abuse?

Another more controversial theme in the Jewish religion is the circumcision. The act of circumcision is largely diffused in the world and is most popular among the entire Hebraic community. It is a symbol of religious identity among the male population. However, in 2012, the Cohort of Cologne in Germany declared circumcision to be illegal. This declaration was accompanied by a great clamour among the European sectors of Judaism, but there was substantial accord among the German population. A recent article discussed this thorny issue from a medical point of view. The authors of this article highlighted the necessity of better research into the consequences of circumcision on sexual behaviour and sexual pleasure in circumcised males [54]. However, although largely accepted, and not only in the Jewish and Muslim environment, it is difficult not to consider male circumcision a sexual mutilation.

7.3.4 Islam

While male circumcision is practised in the Hebraic religions, **female genital mutilations** are often associated with the Islamic traditions, although this terrible form of abuse is not limited to the Muslim religion [55]. The Muslim religion in Islam was founded based on the writings in the Quran, as well as on the teachings of the prophet Muhammad, through the A'hadith text.

The terrible cases of abuse towards women that are often reported on by daily news agencies, particularly in the form of genital mutilation, are not supported by teachings from the **Quran**. In fact, gender discrimination is influenced by the cultural practices over centuries, in addition to the place or nation. The violent practices towards females and the concept of women have changed from Africa to Arabia. Regardless, the degeneration of religion and the misinterpretation of the sacred books continue to be the main causes of abuse against women.

In an interesting study, the factors associated with domestic violence against women in Saudi Arabia were highlighted [56]. There were 2,301 women who participated in this study. The researchers investigated many parameters, including important socio-demographic features. The main results revealed that financial dependency of the female partner and the use of alcohol by the male partner were associated with a greater risk of violent acts towards women [56].

Some studies have also described the situation in sub-Saharan Africa regarding the abuse of child orphans. For example, a review stated that orphans are more exposed to sexual abuse, often in the forms of prostitution or youth marriage. Also in this case, alcohol abuse and poverty could be considered predictive factors of child abuse [57].

Another remarkable aspect of the Muslim religion concerns the controversial role of the veil worn by Muslim women. The role of the veil among Muslim women represents an important issue in some of the European legislations. While some people consider the veil to be a symbol of female submission, others view it as a symbol of cultural and religious identity. Hence, the veil remains the object of many debates and reflections.

7.3.5 Hinduism

A recent campaign against violence towards women showed dramatic pictures representing great female Indian goddesses with facial ecchymosis. It is important to note that more than 68 % of women in India are victims of domestic violence. This aspect reveals a paradox concerning the religious ideals and the actual reality. In the Indian culture, women are simultaneously viewed as both venerable goddesses and as victims of abuse.

Another phenomenon in the Hindu religion regards child marriage in India. This practice represents a great violation of child rights. Statistics show that 50 % of women in the Hindu tradition are married prior to 18 years of age. Child marriage often results in many consequences, including child mortality and domestic violence. Data collected by UNICEF report the main characteristics of child marriage in the rural area of India [58]. Approximately 52.5 % of child marriages occur in the rural areas of India, while 28.2 % of child marriages occur in the urban areas of the country. However, gender disparity is present in both of the areas.

An interesting factor in child marriages concerns the religious affiliation among the Indian people involved in this form of marriage. The median age of marriage in the Jain, Sikh and Christian communities is significantly higher as compared to the average age of marriage in the Hindu and Muslim communities. In these latter communities, the median age is 17.3, demonstrating the strong impact of a specific religious affiliation on the practice of child marriage [58]. This phenomenon is also explained by other characteristics, such as social status and level of education.

Child marriage represents a risk for the health of the child due to the possibility of pregnancy occurring in the female at a very young age. Moreover, the child brides are exposed to domestic violence, isolation and psychological diseases at a greater level than are adult brides.

An interesting article states that the female role in India contrasts with the role of women in sacred scriptures, such as the Vedas. According to the Vedic cultural practices of the past, we can clearly see that the women enjoyed great respect [53]. Hence, in this case, religion is not always directly responsible for various forms of abuse, such as the phenomenon of child brides.

7.3.6 The Cult of Satan

Certainly the media resonance of an abusive priest spreads more quickly and raises greater interest, but sexual violence is also present in minor spiritual contexts such as satanism and demonism.

Satanic cults originate in ancient times and are handed down to Christianity as an evil figure and evil practices. The psychologist **James Hillman** in the book *An Essay on Pan* asserts that iconography and the symbolic features of evil are directly derived from Pan, the Greek god of nature and instinct [59]. **Pan** was described as half-man and half-goat and he was the god of masturbation, rape and unlimited transgression.

In about 1970, Anton LaVey founded the *Church of Satan* and later published the *Satanic Bible*, a text in which any kind of egoism was praised [60]. The Church of Satan underwent multiple divisions giving rise to other groups devoted to the devil cult; they were characterised by rituals involving sexual perverted practices and drug use. In the 1980s, in the United States and Europe the first trials of child sexual abuse crimes in sects took place.

Also in these cases, the satanic phenomenon was examined from both the legal and the psychiatric point of view. Many of the satanic cult members perpetuating the most violent sexual perversions ranging from incestuous rape to cannibalism were reported to be affected by multiple personality disorder [61]. Others, after forensic and psychiatric assessment, showed a fragile, immature personality, a very low level of education and social disadvantages [62]. It is evident that satanism attains much more to brutal criminology and to the dramatic psychopathology of a paraphilic sick sexuality than to the religious field.

Conclusions

The consequences of abuse in religious and spiritual contexts are dramatic and involve and affect the whole life of the victim. In particular, in the continued abused–abusive relationship, victims unconsciously activate the defence mechanism of **identification with the aggressor**. The abused subject introjects the aggressor figure who disappears from external reality but continues to act unconsciously, consolidating the abusive experience as traumatic recollection.

Another psychic mechanism that allows the mental integrity of the abused is **dissociation**. Dissociative phenomena allow the victim to maintain self-functioning and to survive repeated traumas through an evolutionary process in which sorrow, suffering and shame are not verbalised.

Some research also highlights psychobiological deregulations in abused children that alter brain development. Changes pertain to hyperactivation of the Hypothalamus–Pituitary–Adrenal axis, volume reductions in the amygdala and hippocampus, reduced metabolism of the orbitofrontal cortex and reduced structural connectivity of the right hemisphere functions [63–65].

On the other hand, religion and spirituality, from a psychological point of view, also constitute the main coping strategies to face stressful life events [66]. Religious coping can help people to react to individual and collective negative situations such as chronic illness, grief or exposure to a collective trauma such as a war or a natural catastrophe [67]. Religion and faith are significant and useful psychological resources that can literally save the mind and the soul of a subject who is going through a deep crisis.

Therefore, the use of religion and spirituality could be considered a *pharmakos*: it is a remedy for health and safety, but, at the same time, as suggested by the Greek etymology, a dangerous poison when it includes a combination of fanaticism and psychopathology.

References

1. Grier PE, Clark M, Stoner SB (1993) Comparative study of personality traits of female sex offenders. Psychol Rep 73:1378
2. Travin S, Cullen K, Protter B (1990) Female sex offenders: severe victims and victimizers. J Forensic Sci 35:140–150
3. Green R (2002) Is pedophilia a mental disorder? Arch Sex Behav 31:467–471
4. Welldon E (1995) Madre, madonna, prostitute. Centro Scientifico Torinese, Torino
5. Childline (2009) Children talking to ChildLine about sexual abuse. https://www.nspcc.org.uk/Inform/publications/casenotes/clcasenotessexualabuse2_wdf69493.pdf
6. Valcarenghi M (2007) Ho paura di me: Il comportamento sessuale violento. Mondatori, Milano

7. Enquist M, Aronsson H, Ghirlanda S, Jansson L, Jannini EA (2011) Exposure to mother's pregnancy and lactation in infancy is associated with sexual attraction to pregnancy and lactation in adulthood. J Sex Med 8:140–147
8. Petrone L, Rialti S (1998) Le caratteristiche di personalità del pedofilo. In: Giommi R, Perrotta M (eds) Pedofilia. Gli abusi, gli abusati, gli abusanti. Edizioni del Cerro, Firenze
9. Petrone L, Troiano M (2005) E se l'orco fosse lei? Strumenti per l'analisi, la valutazione e la prevenzione dell'abuso al femminile. Franco Angeli, Milano
10. Petrone L, Lamberti E (2011) Pedofilia Rosa - Il Crollo dell'Ultimo Tabù. Magi Edizioni Scientifiche, Roma
11. Senn TE, Carey MP, Vanable PA, Coury-Doniger P, Urban M (2007) Characteristics of sexual abuse in childhood and adolescence influence sexual risk behaviour in adulthood. Arch Sex Behav 36:637–645
12. Knopp FH, Lackey LD (1987) Female sexual abusers: a summary of data from 44 treatment providers. Safety Society, Brandon, VT
13. Araji SK (1997) Sexually aggressive children: coming to understand them. Sage, Thousand Oaks, CA
14. Limoncin E, Carta R, Gravina GL, Carosa E, Ciocca G, Di Sante S, Isidori AM, Lenzi A, Jannini EA (2014) The sexual attraction toward disabilities: a preliminary internet-based study. Int J Impot Res 26(2):51–54
15. Kelly BD (2010) Intellectual disability, mental illness and offending behaviour: forensic cases from early 20th century Ireland. Ir J Med Sci 179:409–416
16. Lindsay WR, Hastings RP, Beech AR (2011) Forensic research in offenders with intellectual and development of disabilities: prevalence and risk assessment. Psychol Crime Law 17:3–7
17. Lunsky Y, Raina P, Jones J (2012) Relationship between prior legal involvement and current crisis for adults with intellectual disability. J Intellect Dev Disabil 37(2):163–168
18. Holland T, Clare IC, Mukhopadhyay T (2002) Prevalence of criminal offending by men and women with intellectual disability and the characteristics of offenders: implications for research and service development. J Intellect Disabil Res 46(Suppl 1):6–20
19. Holland S, Persson P (2011) Intellectual disability in Victorian prison system: characteristics of prisoners with an intellectual disability released from prison in 2003–2006. Psychol Crime Law 17:25–42
20. Raina P, Lunsky Y (2010) A comparison study of adults with intellectual disability and psychiatric disorder with and without forensic involvement. Res Dev Disabil 31:218–223
21. O'Brien G, Taylor JL, Lindsay WR et al (2010) Multicentre study of adults with learning disabilities referred to services for antisocial offending behaviour: demographic, individual, offending and service characteristics. J Learn Disabil Offending Behav 2:5–15
22. Lindasy R, O'Brien G, Carson D et al (2010) Pathways into services for offenders with intellectual disabilities. Crim Justice Behav 37:678–694
23. Finkelhor D (1984) Child sexual abuse: new theory and research. Collier McMillan, London
24. Groth AN (1979) Sexual trauma in the life histories of rapists and child molesters. Victimology 4:10–16
25. Dhawan S, Marshall WL (1996) Sexual abuse histories of sexual offenders. Sex Abuse 8:7–15
26. Hanson RK, Slater S (1988) Sexual victimisation in the history of child sexual abusers. A review. Ann Sex Res 1:485–499
27. Williams LM, Siegel JA, Barnyard VL, Jasinski JL, Gartner KL (1995) Juvenile and adult offending behaviour and other outcomes in a cohort of sexually abused boys: 20 years later. Family Research Laboratory, University of New Hampshire, Durham, NY [reported in Cycle of Sexual Abuse (1996). Report to the Subcommittee on Crime, Committee on the Judiciary, House of Representativeness]
28. Lindsay W, Steptoe L, Haut F (2012) Brief report: the sexual and physical abuse histories of offenders with intellectual disability. J Intellect Disabil Res 56(3):326–331
29. American Psychiatric Association (2013) Diagnostic and statistical manual of mental disorders (DSM-5). American Psychiatric Association, Washington, DC

30. Day K (1997) Sex offenders with learning disabilities. In: Read SG (ed) Psychiatry in learning disability. W. B. Saunders, London, pp 278–306
31. Lunsky Y, Frijters J, Griffiths DM, Watson SL, Williston S (2007) Sexual knowledge and attitudes of men with intellectual disability who sexually offend. J Intellect Dev Disabil 32(2):74–81
32. Griffiths D (2007) Sexuality and people who have intellectual disabilities. In: Brown I, Percy M (eds) A comprehensive guide to intellectual and developmental disabilities. Paul H. Brookes, Baltimore, MD, pp 571–581
33. Michie AM, Lindsay WR, Martin V, Grieve A (2006) A test of counterfeit deviance: a comparison of sexual knowledge in groups of sex offenders with intellectual disability and controls. Sex Abuse 18:271–278
34. Talbot TJ, Langdon PE (2006) A revised sexual knowledge assessment tool for people with intellectual disabilities: is sexual knowledge related to sexual offending behaviour? J Intellect Disabil Res 50(Pt 7):523–531
35. Haaven J, Schlank A (2001) The challenge of treating the sex offenders with developmental disabilities. In: Schlank A (ed) The sexual predator: legal issues, clinical issues, special populations. Civic Research Institute, Kingston, NJ, pp 13-1–13-19
36. Camilleri J, Quinsey V (2011) Appraising the risk of sexual and violent recidivism among intellectual disabled offenders. Psychol Crime Law 17:59–74
37. Gray N, Fitzgerald S, Taylor J, Snowdon RJ (2007) Predicting future reconviction in offenders with intellectual disabilities: the predictive efficacy of the VRAG, PCL-SV and the HCR-20. Psychol Assess 19:474–479
38. Griffiths D, Lunsky Y (2003) Socio-sexual knowledge and attitudes assessment tool-revised (SSKAAT-R), [test and manual]. Stoelting, Wood Dale, IL
39. Dagnan D, Sandhu S (1999) Social comparison, self-esteem and depression in people with intellectual disability. J Intellect Disabil Res 43:372–379
40. Marshall WL, Maric A (1996) Cognitive and emotional components of generalized empathy deficits in child molesters. J Child Sex Abus 5:101–110
41. Cooper AJ (1995) Review of the role of two anti-libidinal drugs in the treatment of sex offenders with mental retardation. Ment Retard 33:42–48
42. Plaud JJ, Plaud DM, Kolstoe PD, Orvedal L (2000) Behavioural treatment of sexually offending behaviour. Ment Health Aspect Dev Disabil 3:54–61
43. Murphy GH, Sinclair N, Hays SJ et al (2010) SOTSEC-ID. Effectiveness of group cognitive behavioural treatment for men with intellectual disabilities at risk of sexual offending. J App Res Intellect Disabil 23:537–551
44. Singh NN, Lancioni GL, Winton ASW, Singh AN, Adkins AD, Singh J (2011) Can adult offenders with intellectual disabilities use mindfulness-based procedures to control their deviant sexual arousal? Psychol Crime Law 17(2):165–179
45. Rosemberg ML, Fenley MA (1991) Violence in America. A public health approach. Oxford University Press, New York, NY
46. Girard R (1972) La Violence et le sacré. Bernard Grasset, Paris
47. Zolla E (1998) Il Dio dell'Ebbrezza. Einaudi, Torino
48. Nietzsche F (2004) La nascita della tragedia. Adelphi, Milano
49. Frawley-O'Dea MG, Goldner V (2007) Predatory priests, silenced victims. The sexual abuse crisis and the Catholic Church. Taylor & Francis, New York, NY
50. Parkinson PN, Oates RK, Jayakody AA (2012) Child sexual abuse in the Anglican Church of Australia. J Child Sex Abus 21(5):553–570
51. Roth F (1970) Il lamento di Portnoy. Bompiani, Milano
52. Meghnagi D (1997) Il padre e la legge. Marsilio, Venezia
53. Zaidi S, Ramarajan S, Qiu R, Raucher M, Chadwick R, Nossier A (2009) Sexual rights and gender roles in a religious context. Int J Gynecol Obstet 106:151–155
54. Merkel R, Putzke H (2013) After Cologne: male circumcision and the law. Parental right, religious liberty or criminal assault? J Med Ethics 39(7):444–449

55. Lawani OL, Onyebuchi AK, Iyoke CA, Okeke NE (2014) Female genital mutilation and efforts to achieve Millennium Development Goals 3, 4, and 5 in southeast Nigeria. Int J Gynaecol Obstet 125(2):125–128
56. Fageeh WMK (2014) Factors associated with domestic violence: a cross-sectional survey among women in Jeddah, Saudi Arabia. BMJ Open 4:e004242
57. Morantza G, Coleb D, Vreemanc R, Ayayad S, Ayukud D, Braitstein P (2013) Child abuse and neglect among orphaned children and youth living in extended families in sub-Saharan Africa: what have we learned from qualitative inquiry? Vulnerable Child Youth Stud 8(4):338–352
58. UNICEF (2012) Child marriage in India. An analysis of available data. http://www.unicef.it
59. Hillman J (2001) Saggio su Pan. Adephi, Milano
60. LaVey AS (1968) La Bibbia di Satana. Arcana, Roma
61. Mulhern S (1994) Satanism, ritual abuse, and multiple personality disorder: a sociohistorical perspective. Int J Clin Exp Hypn 42(4):265–288
62. Birkhoff J, Candelli C, Zeroli S, La Tegola D, Carabellese F (2013) The "Bestie di Satana" murders. J Forensic Sci 58(6):1660–1665
63. Caretti V, Capraro G, Schimenti A (2013) Memorie traumatiche e Mentalizzazione. Astrolabio, Roma
64. White RB, Gilliland RMR (1977) I meccanismi di difesa. Astrolabio, Roma
65. Lingiardi V, Madeddu F (2002) I meccanismi di difesa, Teoria, valutazione, clinica. Raffaello Cortina Editore, Milano
66. Shapiro DL, Levendosky AA (1999) Adolescent survivors of childhood sexual abuse: the mediating role of attachment style and coping in psychological and interpersonal functioning. Child Abuse Negl 23(11):1175–1191
67. Stratta P, Capanna C, Riccardi I, Perugi G, Toni C, Dell'Osso L, Rossi A (2013) Spirituality and religiosity in the aftermath of a natural catastrophe in Italy. J Relig Health 52(3):1029–1037

Index

A
Abuser–abused cycle, 96–97
Adjustment disorders, 10
Aggression/aggressive, 94, 95
Alcohol/other psychoactive substance abuse, 10
Androgen deprivation therapy, 22–29
Antiandrogen cyproterone (CPA), 101
Antiandrogen medroxyprogesterone (MPA), 101
Antidepressant medications, 84
Antigay bullying, 40
Antigay hostility as defense mechanism, 34
Antisocial personality disorder, 10
Anxiety disorders, 10, 75
Appetitive/threatening, 66
Assessment, 2, 9–11
Attention deficit hyperactivity disorder (ADHD), 98

B
Body image and body dissatisfaction, 83
Borderline personality disorder (BPD), 10, 74
Bulimic symptoms, 83

C
Case vignettes, 2, 12–13
Casual sex, 41
Childhood maltreatment, 75
Childhood sexual abuse (CSA), 61–66, 68, 71–73
Christian Churches, 102–103
Cognitive-behavioural treatment (CBT), 101
Coming out, 39
Conduct disorder, 10
Counterfeit deviance, 99
Course, 2, 4, 12
Cyproterone acetate (CPA), 23–27

D
Defence mechanisms, 96
Definition of pedophilia, 2–4
Depressive symptoms, 75
Diagnosis, 73
Diagnostic criteria, 2–5
Discrimination, 49–53, 55, 56
Disgust, 36
Dissociative defense mechanism, 39
Drug and alcohol abuse, 75
Dysthymia and depressive disorders, 10

E
Eating disorders (EDs), 76
Educational climate, 42
Emotion dysregulation, 82–83
Epidemiology, 2, 5–6, 63–64
Etiology, 2, 7–8

F
Familial rejection, 41
Family/social support, 79–80
Female paedophilia, 93, 96
Forensic vs. non-forensic samples, 98

G
Gay bashing, 35
Gender, 4, 5, 78–79
Gender subversions, 34
GnRH analogs, 26, 27

H
Heteronormative bias, 42
Heterosexism, 34
Heterosexist, 42
Hinduism, 104–105
Homonegativity, 33

Homophobia, 33
Homophobic bullying, 40
Hypothalamic–pituitary–adrenal axis (HPA), 80–81, 84

I
Immature, 95
Implicit Association Test/Task (IAT), 35, 66
Impulse control disorders, 10
Individual's own conflicted homosexual feelings, 34
Intellectual disabilities (ID), 97, 99
Internalized antigay prejudice, 38
Internalized homophobia, 38
Islam, 104

J
Judaism, 103

L
Latent, 95
Long-lasting effects, 77

M
Manic/hypomanic episode, 10
Measure of Internalized Sexual Stigma for Lesbians and Gay Men (MISS-LG), 36
Mediators, 73–74
Medroxyprogesterone acetate (MPA), 25–27
Mental health, 53–55, 79
Mental retardation, 10
Methodological issues, 72
Microaggressions of everyday life, 39
Minority stress, 37
Moderators, 73–74, 77–78
Modern Homophobia Scale (MHS), 35

N
Narcissistic personality disorder, 10
Neurobiological systems, 78
Neuroticism, 81

O
Obsessive–compulsive disorder (OCD), 7, 10
Occasional, 95
Onset, 2, 4, 8, 9

P
Paraphilias, 5, 10, 11, 17–19, 21, 24–29
Pedophilia, 1–13
    female, 93, 96
Pedophilic disorder, 1–3, 6,

Perceived stigma, 38
Positive/negative valence, 66
Posttraumatic stress disorder (PTSD), 65, 75
Prevalence data, 94–95
Prevalence rates, 98
Preventative policies and practices, 41
Psychiatric conditions, 67, 73
Psychoform dissociation, 76–77
Psychological mechanisms, 64
Psychopathological conditions, 79
Psychotherapy, 85

R
Regressive, 95
Reparative therapies, 42
Resilience, 41
Revictimization, 80
Risk factor, 72
Romantic/passionate view, 64–65
Rosenberg Self-Esteem Scale, 100

S
Same-sex couples, 39
Satanic cults, 105–106
School climate, 41
Secondary victimization, 42
Selective serotoninergic reuptake inhibitors (SSRIs), 21
Self-schemas, 64–65
Self-stigma, 34–36, 38, 43
Serotonin transporter gene promoter region polymorphism (5HTTLPR), 80
Sex
    offenders, 100
    offense, 18–19
    under influence of alcohol and drugs, 41
Sexual abuse research, 62–63
Sexual abuses, 102
Sexual dysfunction, 64–67, 83–84
Sexual fantasies/urges, 99
Sexual function, 63–64
Sexual harassment behavior, 41
Sexually compulsive behaviors, 39
Sexual minority youths, 40
Sexual prejudice, 34
    evaluation of, 35–36
Silence, 39
Social and legal perspectives, 9
Social context, 79
Social isolation, 39
Socio-Sexual Knowledge and Attitudes Assessment Tool—Revised (SSKAAT-R), 100
Statistical models, 65
Stigma, 49, 50, 53–55

Stressful/traumatic experiences related to same-sex attraction, 39
Suicidal behavior, 41

T
Testosterone, 21–27
Theoretical models, 62
Transphobia, 49–56

V
Victorian Institute of Forensic Medicine (VIFM), 72–73
Violence Risk Appraisal Guide (VRAG), 100

W
World Health Organization, 61

CPSIA information can be obtained at www.ICGtesting.com
Printed in the USA
BVOW11s0055051214

378041BV00003B/6/P

9 783319 067865